Consumer Reports

The Best of Health

Marvin M. Lipman, M.D.,
and the Editors of
Consumer Reports on Health

Updated, December 1999

Manufactured in the United States of America

Consumer Reports Best of Health is published by Consumers Union, the nonprofit organization that publishes CONSUMER REPORTS, the monthly magazine of test reports, product Ratings, and buying guidance. Established in 1936, Consumers Union is chartered under the Not-for-Profit Corporation Law of the State of New York.

The information contained in this book is not intended to substitute for professional or medical advice. Consumers Union disclaims responsibility or liability for any loss that may be incurred as a result of the use or application of any information included in **Consumer Reports Best of Health.** Readers should always consult their physicians or other professionals for treatment and advice.

A SPECIAL PUBLICATION
FROM CONSUMER REPORTS
Director, Special Publications Andrea Scott
Managing Editor Bette LaGow
Project Editor Michael Quincy
Special Publications Staff Robert Markovich,
    Pauline Piekarz, Joyce Childs
Designer Debra Roinestad

CONSUMER REPORTS ON HEALTH
Editor Ronni Sandroff
Managing Editor Ronald Buchheim
Medical Editor Marvin M. Lipman, M.D.
Senior Researcher Christopher Hendel
Dental Adviser Irwin Mandel, D.D.S.
Copy Manager Naomi L. Lipman

CONSUMER REPORTS
Editor Julia Kagan
Executive Editor Eileen Denver
Design Director George Arthur
Managing Art Director Tim LaPalme
Publishing Operations Director Reed Fox
Circulation Director Simon Aronin
Promotion Manager Liz McNamara
Promotion Assistant Maryanne Molnar
Retail Sales & Marketing Geoff Baldwin
Manufacturing Coordinator Steven Schiavone

CONSUMERS UNION
President Rhoda H. Karpatkin
Executive Vice President Joel Gurin

Contents

Preface

Consumer Reports Best of Health is published by Consumers Union, the nonprofit organization that publishes **Consumer Reports on Health**, a monthly newsletter on nutrition, fitness, and medical matters, and CONSUMER REPORTS, the monthly magazine best known for test reports, product Ratings, and buying guidance. CONSUMER REPORTS is also a comprehensive source of unbiased advice about products and services, personal finance, health and nutrition, and other consumer concerns. Since 1936, our mission has been to test products, inform the public, and protect consumers. Our income is derived solely from the sale of CONSUMER REPORTS magazine and our other publications and services, and from nonrestrictive, noncommercial contributions, grants, and fees. We buy all the products we test, just as you do. We accept no ads from companies, nor do we let any company use our reports or Ratings for commercial purposes.

SERVICES FROM CONSUMER REPORTS

CONSUMER REPORTS. Published monthly, CONSUMER REPORTS magazine provides impartial information on brand-name products, services, health, and personal finance. To subscribe (13 issues, including the annual Buying Guide, $26), write to us at P.O. Box 53029, Boulder, Colo. 80322-6356.

CONSUMER REPORTS ON HEALTH. Subscription rates: U.S. only: $24 for 1 year, $39 for 2 years. All other countries add $6 per year. (Canadian subscriptions include Goods and Services Tax, registration No. 127047702.) Phone orders and subscription problems: 800 234-2188.

CONSUMER REPORTS SPECIAL PUBLICATIONS. We publish a series of specialty buying guides sold on newsstands and in bookstores, as well as books on finance, drugs, and other issues of consumer concern.

CONSUMER REPORTS ONLINE. Our web site, *www.ConsumerReports.org*, offers convenient access to our information and advice. Free areas provide useful listings, shopping guidance, product recalls, and sample reports. Site subscribers pay $3.95 a month or $24 a year ($19 for CONSUMER REPORTS subscribers) for unlimited use, including searchable access to more than 40 months' worth of our Ratings, recommendations, and advice; participation in discussion groups; and the current issue.

CONSUMER REPORTS TRAVEL LETTER. Monthly newsletter with travel values. To subscribe (12 issues, $39), write us at P.O. Box 53629, Boulder, Colo. 80322-3629.

ZILLIONS. Bimonthly magazine for kids ages 8 and up. To subscribe (6 issues, $16), write us at P.O. Box 54861, Boulder, Colo. 80322-4861.

CONSUMER REPORTS BY REQUEST. Specially edited reports are available by fax or mail. Call 800 789-3715 for an index of what's available. The index costs $1.

OTHER MEDIA. Information from CONSUMER REPORTS is available on TV and radio around the country, and in columns appearing in more than 500 newspapers.

AUTOMOTIVE INFORMATION. Consumer Reports New Car Price Service. Our reports compare sticker price to dealer's invoice. Call 800 933-5555. **Consumer Reports Used Car Price Service.** Find the market value and reliability data for most 1983 to 1998 cars. Call 800 422-1083. **Consumer Reports Auto Insurance Price Service.** Compare the cost of auto insurance for the coverage you need; find the best price. Now available in Ala., Ariz., Calif., Colo., Conn., Fla., Ga., Idaho, Ill., La., Mich., Minn., Miss., Mo., N.C., Nev., N.J., N.M., N.Y., Ohio, Pa., Tenn., Tex., Utah, Va., Wash., and Wis. Call 800 944-4104.

Introduction

A popular feature of CONSUMER REPORTS magazine is "A Question of Health," a column in which the editors answer questions from readers on a wide variety of health topics. A similar column in the **Consumer Reports on Health** newsletter is "On Your Mind." Most of the contents of *The Best of Health* have been drawn from those two sources.

The Best of Health also includes many "Office Visit" columns, a regular feature in **Consumer Reports on Health,** by Marvin M. Lipman, M.D., Consumers Union's chief medical adviser. These discussions, highly readable and full of practical advice, cover a wide range of health problems. The case histories are taken directly from Dr. Lipman's own medical practice. Irwin D. Mandel, D.D.S., Consumers Union's dental consultant, joins the discussion with an "Office Visit" on bad breath and another that describes ways of evaluating your dentist and, if necessary, finding a new one.

The Best of Health is easy to use. Each major topic is listed alphabetically, with specific problems arranged under the appropriate heading. Following many of the main questions and answers are "Office Visit" columns that discuss the same topic from a different angle and in greater detail.

Simply check the table of contents or consult the index to find the subjects that interest you. You're bound to find some questions (and answers) or some health-topic discussions that affect you, a family member, or a friend. Or read the book straight through. Once you get started, *The Best of Health* is hard to put down.

We think you'll find this book enlightening, entertaining, and a valuable source of reliable medical information. All the information has been carefully checked for accuracy and currency.

Allergies

ALLERGY SHOTS

Q. *I've had chronic nasal congestion and figured it was due to an allergy. After skin tests confirmed my hunch, my ear, nose, and throat doctor started giving me desensitization shots. He said I'll need them for the rest of my life. Is that true?*

A. Probably not. Your allergic sensitivity can eventually fade as you age. Allergy shots should be given only as frequently as needed to control symptoms. Typically, that means once a month, perhaps more during allergy season. If symptoms improve, the interval between shots can be increased.

ANTIHISTAMINES IN ADVANCE?

Q. *Should antihistamines be taken prior to allergy season, before symptoms develop, in order to build up immunity against the onslaught of allergens?*

A. No. Antihistamines have no such "priming" effect. They help to combat allergic symptoms only when allergens (allergy-inducing substances) are present.

NASAL SPRAY EVERY DAY?

Q. *My doctor prescribed* Vancenase AQ *nasal spray for me to use every day to control stuffiness and other allergic reactions. But you have advised not to use nasal products for more than three days. Does that advice apply to my medication?*

A. No. That caution concerned nasal decongestants, such as those containing phenylephrine (*Neo-Synephrine, Nostril*), oxymetazoline (*Afrin, Neo-Synephrine 12 Hour*), or xylometazoline (*Inspire, Otrivin*). Decongestant sprays can actually worsen congestion after a few days. The drug you're taking, beclomethasone (*Beconase AQ, Vancenase AQ*), is a nasal steroid, which controls allergic symptoms by a different mechanism and doesn't cause "rebound congestion." Steroid sprays can sometimes irritate the nasal passages, but that can often be prevented by aiming the nozzle properly or by first using a saline spray.

SULFITES ON THE LABEL

Q. *Why do the labels of wine bottles include the phrase "contains sulfites"? Do sulfites have some harmful effect?*

A. Some people—most of them asthmatics—are allergic to sulfite compounds, which have long been used as preservatives in wines. Federal regulations have required the labeling since 1987.

ALLERGY MEDICATION

Q. *I suffer from hay-fever types of allergies (sneezing, sinus headache, watery eyes) and have found that taking one*

Drixoral *each night helps relieve those symptoms the following day. Should I be concerned that taking this for a long time will cause side effects?*

A. *Drixoral Cold and Allergy,* an over-the-counter drug that's a long-acting combination of the decongestant pseudoephedrine and an antihistamine, has few long-term side effects. Some of the short-term effects, such as sedation, may even lessen with continued use. But by using a fixed-dose combination drug you may be taking more than what is needed to treat your allergy symptoms. If sneezing and watery eyes are your main problem, an antihistamine alone would usually suffice, and the decongestant part of the *Drixoral* would be unnecessary.

ALLERGIC TO MAKEUP?

Q. *I would like to know whether some mascara and eye pencils produce allergic reactions such as puffy eyelids, blurred vision, and burning and itching of the eyes. I suspect that some of the chemical ingredients contained in those products are causing those symptoms.*

A. You may be right. Symptoms of an allergic reaction to eye makeup include red, itchy eyes that tear excessively; the eyelids may also turn red or blotchy and thicken. To find out whether your problem is an allergy, stop using cosmetics around your eyes for a few weeks; if it is an allergic response, your symptoms should clear up. Any chemical substance that might come near your eyes, including shampoo, hand cream, or nail polish, should be suspect as well. Lanolin, preservatives, fragrances, formaldehyde, and other ingredients can cause allergic or hypersensitivity reactions.

If your symptoms don't go away, see your doctor. But if the problem does clear up, you can then carefully reintroduce your cosmetics, one product per week, to find out which one may be causing the problem. If necessary, an allergist can test you to determine exactly what you're reacting to.

Alzheimer's disease

ALUMINUM AND ANTACIDS

Q. *I've heard that aluminum might cause Alzheimer's disease and other problems. So is aluminum hydroxide really a safe antacid?*

A. There's no convincing scientific evidence that aluminum ingested from antacids or any other source contributes to Alzheimer's and other dementias.

People with normal kidney function excrete virtually all the aluminum absorbed into the body. But older people (who may have decreased kidney function) and people with known kidney disease tend to retain aluminum within the body. Although that hasn't been shown to cause any harm in these individuals, they should use antacids containing aluminum only on a physician's advice.

Aluminum can contribute to health problems in some persons. For instance, aluminum-related bone disease has occurred in kidney patients on long-term hemodialysis. As a result, dialysis fluids are now more rigorously purified, and physicians try to avoid aluminum compounds—or at least use smaller amounts—in treating kidney disease.

IBUPROFEN FOR ALZHEIMER'S AND THE HEART?

Q. *My doctor has me taking 81 mg of aspirin a day to cut the risk of heart attack and stroke. Would an equivalent amount of ibuprofen do the job? A preliminary study of long-term ibuprofen use showed it delayed Alzheimer's disease, and I'd like to have a shot at preventing all three conditions with one pill.*

A. Ibuprofen (*Advil, Motrin-IB*) doesn't have anywhere near the anti-clotting effect of aspirin, so it won't help prevent heart attack or stroke. And it's premature to take ibuprofen or other nonsteroidal anti-inflammatory drugs in hopes of warding off Alzheimer's—especially since regular use of those drugs can pose significant risks.

✚ *Office Visit*

CARING FOR THE CAREGIVER

I still make house calls. OK, not that many, and usually only when the patient is bedridden and can't easily get to my office or the emergency room. One such patient is a 78-year-old former car dealer who suffered a massive stroke some 15 years ago. The stroke caused complete paralysis of his left arm and leg, loss of speech, and abrupt overall mental decline. I see him at his home two or three times a year.

But this column is not about him, it's about his wife. Now age 68, she has devoted a substantial portion of her life to caring for her invalid husband. "I could have put him in a nursing home years ago," she once told me. "But I couldn't bear the thought of someone else taking care of him. If the situation were reversed, I know he'd do the same for me."

She's fortunate that their finances permit her to live out that decision. But the years of intensive hands-on care have had more than a monetary cost. Hospital paraphernalia has taken over what was once their living room. She spends long days tending to his needs and many sleepless nights answering his calls for assistance. In addition to constant worry and frayed nerves, she has developed symptoms of heart disease and chronic diarrhea. In many ways, she's become sicker than her husband.

THE STRESS OF CAREGIVING

Her predicament is far from unique. Similar stories are played out in some 22 million households in the U.S. today—nearly triple the number of just over a decade ago. About three-fourths of the caregivers are women, usually caring for their husbands or, less often, a parent.

The constant burden on the caregiver can result in a great deal of psychological distress—including anxiety, depression, and crushing guilt. More difficult still may be the emotional stress of watching a loved one deteriorate physically and mentally.

Then there's the financial crunch. Many people lack long-term insurance for a chronic debilitating condition. With limited Medicare coverage and seemingly limitless expenses, few people in such a situation can withstand the economic pressure indefinitely.

Some evidence suggests that all the compounded stress may contribute to the development of physical illness. Certainly, the relentless physical demands of caring for an aging or ailing relative can be exhausting as well. Especially for an older caregiver, lifting, bathing, toileting, and dressing a near-helpless adult can lead to sprains and strains, even falls and fractures.

GETTING HELP

Sooner or later, most caregivers realize they need help. A good way to start tracking down resources is to contact a social worker in a local hospital or call your state or county health department—specifically, the agency on aging or the division responsible for social services. Those sources can point you toward helpful programs and groups. Some agencies, for example, offer financial advice, assistance with tax and Medicare forms, and help in locating special-needs housing. They may also administer services that provide transportation and meals.

Often, a caregiver's most pressing need is simply some rest or a chance to get away from all the responsibilities for a few days. Many programs can now satisfy that need, including "respite" care programs offered by nursing homes and other for-profit agencies. In addition, less expensive adult day-care programs are increasingly offered by community organizations such as local Y's, churches, and synagogues. Depending on sponsorship, the cost may be based on a sliding scale or may even be free. However, because there's often little regulatory oversight, you have to scrutinize such programs before relinquishing care of your loved one for even a few hours. Visit in advance and ask lots of questions.

Caregivers who need more than an occasional hand may have to hire an aide to help out in their home regularly. To find such an aide, you can either hire someone yourself or rely on a home health agency. In either case, don't hesitate to shop around until you find a person you like and trust.

At some point, it just may not be feasible to continue caring for a chronically ill or disabled loved one at home. Then you'll want to look into institutional care. The options range from residence centers for mobile patients who need limited assistance to nursing homes for bedridden patients who need continual medical and personal care. You can get a list of licensed facilities from your local agency on aging. Or get recommendations from friends or professionals.

To function as an effective caregiver, it's important to look after your own needs as well. Be sure to let family members and friends know that you'd appreciate their help from time to time. Consider joining a caregiver support group, if there's one in your community. And give yourself a break: Go on a much-needed vacation—even if only for a few days. You've got to take good care of yourself if you're going to take care of someone else.

Arthritis and joint and muscle disorders

ARTHRITIS AND COD-LIVER OIL

Q. *I read in the book* Arthritis and Common Sense *that cod-liver oil can help treat arthritis. Can it really?*

A. No. The author of that popular book, Dale Alexander, claimed that the basic cause of arthritis is dry joints and that dietary oils, particularly cod-liver oil, relieve arthritis by lubricating the joints. That's wrong.

There's never any "oil" in the joints, regardless of what you eat; the lubricating fluid, which resembles blood plasma, is secreted by the tissue lining the joints. Only in the Land of Oz can the joints be oiled.

ARTHRITIS AND HEART ATTACK

Q. *To treat my arthritis, I take* Trilisate, *which my doctor says is in the aspirin family. Since aspirin can help prevent heart attacks, would the drug I'm taking offer some protection as well?*

A. No. Aspirin is believed to cut the risk of heart attack by making the blood less likely to clot. *Trilisate* (choline and magnesium salicylates) has no such effect. While other non-steroidal anti-inflammatory drugs—such as ibuprofen (*Advil, Motrin-IB*), naproxen (*Aleve, Naprosyn*), and oxaprozin (*Daypro*)—can inhibit clotting somewhat, their blood-thinning effect is far less pronounced than that of aspirin. And only aspirin has been shown to reduce the risk of heart attack. (The other drugs, however, have not been adequately studied for this effect.)

BURSITIS OF THE HIP

Q. *How common is bursitis of the hip, and what can be done about it? I had my first siege 10 months ago, and although* Feldene *helped a lot, the bursitis has not disappeared entirely.*

A. Although bursitis most often affects the shoulder, bursitis of the hip is also quite common. Knees and elbows are also vulnerable. At all those joints, tiny sacs called bursae are located between the tendon and bone. When a bursa becomes inflamed, often because of injury or overuse, the joint aches.

Standard treatment consists of rest and oral anti-inflammatory medication such as naproxen *(Aleve, Naprosyn)*. Sometimes injections of a corticosteroid drug directly into the bursa can be helpful. The inflammation and pain usually pass with time but can recur. In rare instances, surgery may be necessary.

CALCIUM DEPOSITS

Q. *I have calcium deposits on the tendons in my shoulder. My doctor has prescribed anti-inflammatory drugs and tells me the deposits can be removed only by surgery. Is there any alternative? I also wonder if taking calcium supplements affects the condition.*

A. Calcium deposits tend to form on a tendon that has been inflamed for some time. Such deposits have nothing to do with the calcium you ingest, either in food or in supplements.

Anti-inflammatory medications are able to relieve the discomfort, but only temporarily. Graduated exercises, heat or cold treatments, and sometimes corticosteroid injections can also help. Surgery is usually reserved for severe cases, such as a "frozen" shoulder that doesn't respond to exercise therapy.

CRACKED KNUCKLES

Q. *I have a habit of cracking my knuckles. Is that really harmful?*

A. The answer's still not certain. One study has found that habitual knuckle crackers are more likely to have swollen hands and a weaker grip. The researchers concluded that the habit "results in functional hand impairment." It's also possible that such impairment simply results from the loose joints that let people crack knuckles in the first place. To play it safe, heed your mother's advice and stop cracking your knuckles.

FIBROMYALGIA: WHAT DOES IT MEAN?

Q. *I have been diagnosed as having fibromyalgia, which comes and goes. I would appreciate an explanation of what it is and whether it is curable or controllable.*

A. Fibromyalgia, also known as fibrositis or fibromyositis, refers to a disorder of unknown cause that is characterized by recurrent pain in the joints, muscles, or tendons. Often small, specific areas called "trigger points" are tender to the touch. Physical strain and cold or damp weather can make the disorder worse. Frequently, the pain is associated with other symptoms, such as insomnia, fatigue, or anxiety. Laboratory tests are usually normal. There are several treatments: physiotherapy, warm or cold compresses, anti-inflammatory medication, and sometimes an anesthetic or cortisone injected directly into the trigger points. The symptoms can wax and wane over many years.

GOLD FOR ARTHRITIS

Q. *For the past six months, I've had weekly injections of gold, which have helped my rheumatoid arthritis. Now my physician has recommended a maintenance injection every four or five weeks for the rest of my life. What are the long-range risks?*

A. Mainly skin rashes, mouth ulcers, and damage to the kidneys or bone marrow, where blood cells are manufactured. Any side effects of gold injections will usually develop during the first few months of treatment, but they can surface during the maintenance period as well. So you'll need a blood count and urine test before each injection.

A possible alternative is auranofin (*Ridaura*), an oral gold preparation. The oral form carries its own side effects and may not be as effective as injections.

Gold therapy has largely been replaced by methotrexate *(Rheumatrex)* and newer medications.

GOUT AND THE DIET

Q. *In addition to taking medication for gout, I also avoid foods high in purine—such as animal organs, herring, mushrooms, sardines, and spinach. I've been told my list of purine-containing foods is incomplete. What others should I avoid?*

A. Many other foods contain purines, notably anchovies, goose, mussels, scallops, yeast, and meat derivatives such as soup stock and gravy. But avoiding purine-containing foods may not be as necessary as it was once thought to be.

Gout is a heritable disease marked by an excess of uric acid in the blood. Severe dietary restriction for people with gout can indeed decrease blood levels of uric acid somewhat. However, today's medications, especially allopurinol (*Lopurin, Zyloprim*), can do the job much better. So moderation in diet rather than avoidance of certain foods is sufficient for most people with gout.

Alcohol, however, is one dietary item that should be restricted, since it may trigger an acute attack of gout.

PSEUDO-GOUT: WHAT IS IT?

Q. *A few months ago I came down with an ailment the medical people refer to as pseudo-gout. What in the world do I have?*

A. You have an illness known as chondrocalcinosis, characterized by painful, stiff joints caused by the buildup of calcium salts in the cartilage. Much less common than regular gout, pseudo-gout affects both men and women equally (gout affects mostly men) and causes attacks of pain that can be less predictable than those of gout. Like gout, pseudo-gout has no cure. Acute attacks can be controlled by colchicine—an anti-inflammatory drug that is specific for gout and pseudo-gout—or by using other anti-inflammatory drugs such as ibuprofen. The latter can also be used in long-term maintenance for those afflicted with repeat episodes.

MUSCLE CRAMPS

Q. *As I've grown older, I've started getting muscle cramps. What can I do about them?*

A. For most cramps, stretch. If a spasm strikes the calf (by far the most common cramp site), pull the front of the foot up toward the knee. Since cramps usually result from muscle fatigue, you may be able to prevent such spasms by gently stretching before you exercise your calves. Stand a few feet from a wall, brace yourself against the wall with your hands, and lean forward, keeping your heels on the ground until you feel a pull in your calves. This maneuver before bedtime can also help prevent unexplained nighttime spasms.

If the cause isn't muscle fatigue, your physician may find

other, possibly treatable causes. These can include circulatory problems, hyperventilation, an underactive thyroid, and low blood levels of calcium or (rarely) magnesium.

POTATOES AND ARTHRITIS

Q. *Is it true that toxins in potatoes and other plants of the nightshade family—including tomatoes, peppers, and egg-plant—can exacerbate or even cause arthritis in some people?*

A. There's no scientific evidence to support that old folk legend. If it were true, populations that eat lots of potatoes would presumably have a higher incidence of arthritis. Epidemiological studies have shown that they don't.

RUB IT IN

Q. *What is it about* BenGay *that helps relieve the pain of arthritis?*

A. *BenGay,* like other muscle-ache and arthritis rubs, provides relief by acting as a counterirritant. It produces a mild local inflammation that crowds out pain messages from nearby muscles and joints. Arthritis rubs also create heat by increasing blood flow to the area; because of the risk of a burn, they should never be used together with a heating pad.

Asthma and lung problems

BLOOD CLOTS IN THE LUNG

Q. *Four weeks after a hysterectomy, my 62-year-old mother died suddenly due to pulmonary emboli, or blood clots in her lung. Should my sisters and I worry that this could happen to us after surgery?*

A. That depends. Susceptibility to pulmonary embolism, which generally develops only after surgery or prolonged bed rest, is not inherited directly. However, two risk factors for the condition—obesity and severe varicose veins—do run in families. Other risk factors include heart failure, certain cancers, and a history of phlebitis (inflamed veins).

People predisposed to pulmonary embolism may receive anticlotting medication after they've undergone abdominal, pelvic, or certain orthopedic operations—or if they'll be bedridden for a long time.

GOOD MOVES FOR ASTHMATICS

Q. *I'm considering a change of climate to help relieve my asthma. I've heard that the dry air of the desert Southwest is beneficial, but also that salty sea air can help. Can you clear up this contradiction?*

A. The best locale for asthma sufferers is one that's free of pollutants, airborne allergens, and frigid weather. Traditionally, asthmatics migrated to Arizona for its warm, dry climate, although the benefit came primarily from cleaner air and lower pollen counts. As Arizona cities have grown, however, the environment there has become less favorable for asthmatics. Sea air has no effect on asthma.

CHEST CONGESTION

Q. *I often have congestion in my nose, ears, and chest. What over-the-counter drugs would you recommend to loosen this congestion in my chest so I can cough it up and spit it out?*

A. The only FDA-approved expectorant for loosening phlegm is guaifenesin. It's found in *Breonesin* tablets, plain *Robitussin* syrup, *Scot-Tussin* syrup, and other over-the-counter products.

However, an expectorant doesn't address the underlying problem, and therefore should be used only occasionally. You may have a chronic problem in your sinuses or bronchial airways. You should be evaluated by a physician for allergies or any other problem that might cause recurrent congestion.

Back pain

DISK DECISION

Q. *Because of a herniated disk, I've been suffering from lower-back pain that radiates to my leg. Is surgery usually necessary, or could other treatment relieve the pain?*

A. Conservative treatment, including limited bed rest, physical therapy, and anti-inflammatory drugs, is often successful in relieving pain from a herniated, or "slipped," disk. Unless the pain or numbness is severe or nerve function is impaired to the point of weakness of your leg muscles, you should try those alternatives for two to three months before resorting to more invasive techniques such as local cortisone injections or surgery.

PUSH-UPS AND BAD BACKS

Q. *I've read that anyone with a "bad back" should not do push-ups. I've never experienced any back problems that I could attribute to push-ups, but now I am concerned. Please elaborate.*

A. Done correctly, push-ups shouldn't harm your back at all. The key is to keep your upper body straight as you push up, whether pivoting from your toes (the classic position) or from your knees (the "modified" push-up). If you arch your back, you'll strain it. That's a common mistake, so people who have had back problems should probably skip push-ups.

A DEVICE FOR TREATING PAIN

Q. *My orthopedist wants me to try a device called a TENS unit to relieve my severe lower-back pain. Is this therapy beneficial, or could it actually harm the nerves?*

A. TENS (transcutaneous electrical nerve stimulation) has been used to treat pain for many years. The battery-powered unit delivers low-voltage pulses through electrodes placed on the skin over the painful area. This low-energy nerve stimulation is believed to interfere with the transmission of pain sensation from the affected area to the brain. About the size of a deck of playing cards, the units are simple to use at home, and there's no evidence that they cause any harm. A TENS unit costs around $100 a month to rent, or $400 to $650 to buy.

TENS provides pain relief for up to 60 percent of patients who use it. When successful, the treatment may eliminate or lessen the need for medication, but the effects of electrical stimulation appear to weaken over time. TENS is often not very effective in relieving severe pain.

Bladder and urinary problems

CANCEROUS BLADDER POLYPS

Q. *My urologist found bladder polyps when he did a cystoscopy on me. After removing them, he said they were cancerous but "low-grade, superficial, and noninvasive." What causes malignant bladder polyps?*

A. Occasionally, a specific carcinogen can be pinpointed as the cause of malignant polyps. The main culprits are cigarette smoking and occupational exposure to aromatic amines, compounds used in many manufacturing and chemical processes. In most cases, however, there's no identifiable cause.

Malignant bladder polyps range from slow-growing, noninvasive tumors to aggressive cancers that rapidly invade the bladder wall. Bladder polyps can also turn out to be benign. In either case, the most effective treatment is removal of the polyps through a cystoscope, a lighted tube inserted into the bladder. After removal of a malignant polyp, the bladder should be reinspected cystoscopically every three to six months for several years. A chemical can also be instilled directly into the bladder to inhibit the development of additional polyps.

INTERSTITIAL CYSTITIS

Q. *What can you tell me about interstitial cystitis? I know it resembles a urinary-tract infection, but it's not an infection.*

A. You're right. Interstitial cystitis is a bladder inflammation, but infection is not to blame. Like a urinary-tract infection, the disease can provoke frequent, urgent urination. Unlike an infection, it often causes pain that is actually relieved by urination.

No one knows what causes interstitial cystitis, and diagnosis can be difficult. There is no cure, so treatment focuses on symptoms. Many approaches have been tried, including distending the bladder with fluid; infusing the bladder with a chemical called DMSO (*Rimso-50*); and giving oral medications such as pentosan (*Elmiron*), the antidepressant amitriptyline (*Elavil*), and various muscle relaxants for the bladder. None has worked consistently.

In one study, patients who didn't have severe pain gradually stretched their bladder by resisting the urge to urinate frequently. Each month, they increased the interval between trips to the bathroom by 15 to 30 minutes. After three months, 15 of the 21 patients reported at least a 50 percent reduction in the urgency and frequency of urination.

Since the disorder often defies medical therapy, patients

have formed a self-help group: The Interstitial Cystitis Association (800 HELP-ICA or 301 610-5300; *(www.ichelp.com)*.

LONG-TERM DIURETICS

Q. *I take a diuretic medication every day. Does the drug lose its effectiveness or cause any harm when taken for many years?*

A. No. Diuretics (drugs that increase urine output) are an effective long-term therapy for hypertension and other disorders. Long-term use doesn't cause harm, although it can result in a low blood-potassium level, which can damage the kidneys.

RESTLESS NIGHTS

Q. *For the past couple of years, an aching fullness in my bladder has prompted me to get up as many as three to four times a night to urinate. I do not experience the same problem during the day. I am 25 years old, female, and otherwise in good health. Do I need to see a doctor?*

A. Not necessarily. First, try drinking less fluid with dinner and during the evening. In particular, refrain from alcohol, which is a diuretic. But if these simple measures don't work, see your doctor. Your "nocturia" could be due to an enlarged pelvic structure pressing on the bladder when you lie down, the nighttime release of daytime water retention, or a kidney disorder.

Blood pressure

DIURETICS IN THE DESERT

Q. *My sister's physician put her on a daily diuretic to treat hypertension. She'll be taking a trip to the desert soon. Should she use salt tablets to prevent dehydration?*

A. No. If the diuretic isn't causing excessive water loss now, dehydration from the heat shouldn't be a problem. Salt tablets might make the body retain water, but that's exactly what the diuretic is supposed to prevent. Your sister should just drink plenty of water to replace what she sweats away.

HEAT AND BLOOD PRESSURE

Q. *Does using a* Jacuzzi *or* sauna *elevate blood pressure in people who already have hypertension?*

A. No. In fact, high ambient temperature typically causes blood pressure to drop as blood vessels dilate in order to keep body temperature constant. That drop in blood pressure can cause you to faint, especially if you're already taking anti-hypertensive medication.

LOW BLOOD PRESSURE

Q. *Recently I tried to donate blood for the first time and was turned away because my blood pressure was too low (80 over 60 that morning). I'm 52 years old and, as far as I know, in good health. I eat a balanced diet and I exercise almost every day. But my blood pressure is usually only about 100 over 70. Should I be worried about that low level?*

A. On the contrary, you should ask for a rebate on your life insurance premium! If you feel healthy, having a relatively low blood pressure like yours is good for the cardiovascular system, since it puts less stress on the blood vessels. If you were not in such good health, low blood pressure could indicate a disorder such as coronary heart disease or low blood volume due to blood loss. The only reason why low pressure would disqualify you as a donor is that the additional lowering due to losing a pint of blood could conceivably cause a fainting spell.

SAFE WITH NORMAL BLOOD PRESSURE?

Q. *I'm 63 years old and in fine health as far as I know. For years my blood pressure has been in the neighborhood of 118/85, which I understand is quite good. If my blood pressure stays down, am I unlikely to experience a heart attack or stroke?*

A. Normal blood pressure is definitely an advantage, but it won't protect you completely. High blood pressure is only one of several risk factors for cardiovascular disease. Others include smoking, high blood cholesterol, lack of exercise, heredity, and diabetes. Nevertheless, recent studies have suggested that even mild elevations of blood pressure increase your risk of problems. That's why it's important to keep track of your pressure, even if it hasn't been high to date.

THE OTHER HYPERTENSION

Q. *What would cause an increase in a 70-year-old's systolic, or upper, blood-pressure reading while the diastolic pressure remains normal? How serious a problem is this?*

A. The stiffening of the arteries that typically occurs with advancing age can cause systolic blood pressure (the pressure in the arteries when the heart contracts) to rise above normal without affecting diastolic pressure (the pressure between contractions). An overactive thyroid or anemia can often produce the same effect. Temporary systolic blood-pressure hikes may result from exercise, stress, or excitement.

Unless extreme, increases in systolic blood pressure probably pose less risk than diastolic hypertension. Many doctors believe borderline systolic hypertension does not require treatment. Elevations above 160 mm Hg, however, should be treated with antihypertensive medication.

Calcium

KIDNEY STONES AND CALCIUM

Q. *My 27-year-old daughter has had surgery twice for kidney stones. Her doctor told her to eliminate high-calcium foods from her diet. My concern is that a low-calcium diet will put her at high risk for osteoporosis. Would you comment?*

A. A low-calcium diet can increase the risk of osteoporosis, an abnormal loss of bone that can lead to fractures in later years. Your daughter's chances of avoiding osteoporosis will improve if she exercises regularly, doesn't smoke, and avoids heavy intake of alcohol and caffeine. There is evidence that low-calcium diets can increase the frequency of kidney stones whereas high-calcium diets can do the opposite. This seeming paradox may have to do with the effect of dietary calcium in preventing the absorption of oxalates from the intestine.

TUMS FOR THE BONES

Q. *My doctor told me to take* Tums, *which is calcium carbonate, as an inexpensive alternative to calcium pills. However, the bottle warns against taking the maximum dose for more than two weeks. Is it safe to take* Tums *indefinitely?*

A. Yes, if you're just taking the modest dose needed as a supplement. The warning on the *Tums* bottle refers to its use as an antacid: Prolonged need for antacids should be evaluated by a doctor. Moreover, large amounts of supplemental calcium—such as the maximum dose of 16 tablets a day for indigestion—can cause constipation, abdominal pain, and kidney stones if taken over a long period.

CALCIUM SOURCES

An adequate calcium intake is essential for warding off the fragile-bone disease osteoporosis. It's a good idea to get as much of that calcium as you can from dietary sources—primarily reduced-fat dairy products and calcium-fortified products such as orange juice. But many people will also need to turn to supplements, which can be a bewildering task. Here are answers to some of the most commonly asked questions about calcium supplements.

How much should I take? Postmenopausal women who are receiving any kind of bone therapy, including estrogen, nasal calcitonin *(Miacalcin Nasal Spray),* and alendronate *(Fosamax),* should get 1,200 milligrams of calcium a day; those who aren't should aim for 1,500 milligrams. Other adults need about 1,000 milligrams up to age 50, 1,200 milligrams from age 50 to 65, and 1,500 milligrams over 65. If you need supplements, take only the amount of calcium required to reach the recommended level. For best absorption, don't take more than 500 milligrams at a time; if you need to take more than that, split up your dose.

How can I tell how much calcium is in a certain supplement? Read the label very carefully. Calcium comes in various compounds, such as calcium carbonate, calcium citrate, calcium gluconate, and others. But only the calcium element itself counts. So ignore how much of the total calcium compound is in each pill; instead, look for the amount of "elemental" calcium.

Which calcium compound is best? The various compounds differ mainly in the amount of elemental calcium they supply. The more calcium you get from a particular compound, the fewer pills you'll have to take. Calcium carbonate—which is also the active ingredient in certain antacid tablets, such as *Tums* and *Rolaids Calcium Rich*—is the most concentrated form of calcium and usually the cheapest, so it's generally the best choice.

When should I take calcium pills? Calcium-carbonate supplements are generally somewhat better absorbed when they're taken with a meal or shortly afterward, although it probably doesn't really matter all that much.

Should I be concerned about potential drug interactions? Calcium pills may interfere with the absorption of various medications—including iron supplements as well as certain prescription drugs, such as tetracycline antibiotics and the osteoporosis medication alendronate *(Fosamax)*. Check with your doctor or pharmacist. If a medication you're taking is affected by calcium supplements, you'll probably need to put at least an hour and a half between the drug and the calcium.

Conversely, certain other medications such as corticosteroids tend to impair the absorption of calcium, whether from pills or from food. People who are taking an extended course of such treatment are therefore at increased risk of developing osteoporosis and should consult their physician about appropriate treatment options. They may need to take more calcium than is normally recommended for someone their age, or their doctor may prescribe medication to counter bone loss.

What about the risk of food interactions? The substances known as phytates, which are found in wheat bran, soybeans, and legumes, can inhibit the absorption of calcium from supplements. If you're eating a meal rich in those foods, take your calcium supplements at a different time—or take a little extra calcium to compensate. The oxalates found in certain green leafy vegetables, including rhubarb, spinach, and Swiss chard, tend to block the absorption of calcium *from those foods,* whether cooked or raw, but they won't affect the amount absorbed from other foods or from supplements.

Should I take other nutrients with my calcium? Your body needs vitamin D to maximize calcium absorption. If you're over 50, you may need a daily vitamin-D supplement—especially if you don't drink fortified milk or eat fatty fish, and you seldom get out in the sun. (If you're at high risk for osteoporosis, talk to your doctor about being tested for a low level of vitamin D.)

Small quantities of the trace minerals magnesium, manganese, and zinc also help the body utilize calcium. But the average American diet provides sufficient amounts for that purpose.

What's the risk of lead contamination? While calcium supplements can contain traces of lead, the risk is low and outweighed by the clear benefit against osteoporosis in people who need extra calcium. Still, the less lead the better, which is why Consumers Union has urged the FDA to require manufacturers to minimize the lead content of their calcium pills.

No one type of calcium compound appears to have a consistently higher lead level than the others. However, natural sources of calcium, such as bonemeal and dolomite, are subject to unpredictable environmental contamination, so they're best avoided.

CALCIUM AND LACTOSE

Q. *I'm a 33-year-old man who can't digest lactose. Since I can't drink milk, I'm concerned that I don't get enough calcium in my diet. So I take a 500-milligram supplement twice a day. Is that necessary?*

A. It's a good idea to get 1,000 milligrams of calcium every day, but you should be able to get that without supplements. One way is to consume milk products with the help of pills containing the digestive enzyme lactase, such as *LactAid* or *Lactrase*. Or you could drink a lactose-reduced milk. Buttermilk and yogurt probably wouldn't trouble you either. Nondairy sources of calcium include broccoli, greens (except spinach), kale, legumes (dried beans, peas, and lentils), and canned sardines and salmon.

CALCIUM ABSORPTION

Q. *I have osteoporosis and need to take supplemental calcium. I also eat lots of whole grains, but recently I've read that the phytic acid in them interferes with the absorption of calcium. Is that true?*

A. The phytates found in wheat bran, soybeans, and legumes can inhibit absorption of calcium from supplements. If you're eating a meal rich in those foods, take your calcium supplements at a different time—or take a little extra calcium to compensate.

Cardiovascular disorders

ACCURATE ANGIOGRAM

Q. *Before I started a strenuous exercise program, my doctor ordered an exercise stress test to check my heart, even though I have no symptoms of coronary heart disease. That test was inconclusive, so I had a thallium stress test, which indicated some coronary disease. To confirm that finding, I underwent angiography, which found no sign of disease. Which test should I believe?*

A. Angiography. This procedure, in which the coronary arteries are injected with dye and examined by X-ray, is the most accurate test for blocked coronary arteries. The two stress tests are safer and less expensive than angiography, which is why they're generally done first. However, it is possible for those stress tests to turn up positive when there's actually nothing wrong.

ASPIRIN, TIA, AND ULCERS

Q. *Several years ago, I experienced a transient ischemic attack (TIA), which my physician said indicates a risk of stroke. As a precaution, he recommended aspirin therapy to reduce the chance of blood clots. After an episode of stomach bleeding, attributed to aspirin's effect on a possible ulcer condition, I turned to Ecotrin, a coated aspirin. Should I stop using any kind of aspirin?*

A. Probably not. Aspirin coated with an acid-resistant shell (*Ecotrin* and generic versions) should dissolve after leaving the stomach and thus cause less irritation than uncoated aspirin. It offers the anticlotting benefits of aspirin, with less gastrointestinal risk. Those benefits are important after a TIA, in which blood flow to the brain is temporarily interrupted.

But considering your history of gastrointestinal bleeding from aspirin, you should have blood counts every couple of months. You can also visually check your stool for signs of internal bleeding (which turns the stool black).

For ordinary pain relief, people with a history of ulcers are usually better off taking acetaminophen.

ATYPICAL ANGINA?

Q. *I've read that angina, the type of chest pain that signals coronary heart disease, is usually brought on by exercise and relieved by rest. I sometimes experience chest discomfort while I'm resting but never while I'm exercising. Could that discomfort still be angina?*

A. It's unlikely. But an uncommon form of coronary disease can cause angina when you're resting or asleep—due to arterial spasm, not blockage. To rule out that possibility, your physician could have you wear a heart monitor for 24 hours. You should also have a treadmill exercise test, even though you haven't noticed the pain while exercising.

If those tests find no sign of coronary disease, your physician will investigate other possible causes of your discomfort. It's most likely to be a temporary problem, such as heartburn or muscle spasms. Occasionally, however, the discomfort reflects a chronic disorder, such as a hiatal hernia or gallbladder disease.

BLOCKED BUNDLE BRANCH

Q. *I'm a 50-year-old male with a "right bundle branch block." Is that cause for concern?*

A. Not necessarily. The bundle branches are fibers within the heart muscle that transmit nerve impulses, causing the right and left ventricles to contract and pump blood into the arteries. Occasionally, transmission in one of the bundles becomes blocked, probably due to a clot in a tiny blood vessel feeding the bundle. The affected ventricle then contracts later than the other ventricle; this shows up as a characteristic pattern on an electrocardiogram. There are usually no symptoms, and there's no treatment.

A blocked bundle branch, particularly on the left, does increase the risk of subsequent heart attack somewhat. That risk is compounded by the presence of other risk factors for coronary heart disease: high blood-cholesterol levels, hypertension, male gender, diabetes, age, smoking, and a family history of coronary heart disease before age 55.

HEART PALPITATIONS

Q. *I'm 62 and have had heart palpitations for years. What can you tell me about them?*

A. "Palpitations" is a nonmedical term for any heart rhythm that feels abnormal. That can include extra beats, dropped beats, forceful beats, rapid beats, or irregular beats. For proper diagnosis, the abnormality must first be "captured" on an electrocardiogram or on a 24-hour heartbeat recording. Palpitations can be caused by emotional stress, an overactive thyroid, certain medications, or diseases of the coronary arteries, heart muscle, or heart valves. Sometimes, there's no detectable cause.

At some point soon, you probably should have your palpitations checked, but first try eliminating a few things on your own—caffeine (coffee, tea, cocoa, chocolate, soda), nasal decongestants, appetite suppressants—and see if it makes a difference.

MAGNESIUM AND THE HEART

Q. *What does a low level of magnesium have to do with abnormal heartbeats?*

A. Too little magnesium in the blood, an uncommon condition that is sometimes caused by chronic diarrhea or excessive alcohol intake, can lead to a type of abnormal heart rhythm known as ventricular tachycardia, a life-threatening event. Supplemental magnesium can correct the problem. However, since too much magnesium can also adversely affect the heart, magnesium blood levels must be monitored closely.

MITRAL VALVE PROLAPSE

Q. *I am in my mid-thirties. A few years ago I was diagnosed as having a heart condition called mitral valve prolapse. What exactly is it, and does it make jogging or other exercise risky?*

A. Mitral valve prolapse (MVP), which seems to run in families, now appears to be more common than doctors previously realized, but is usually a harmless condition. It involves a ballooning of the heart's mitral valve leaflets or flaps, which control blood flow between the two left chambers of the heart. Physicians suspect MVP when they hear a certain type of heart murmur or a clicking sound through the stethoscope.

For the vast majority of people with MVP, the only health risk is a mitral valve infection following dental procedures that involve bleeding. If you have MVP, it is very important to let your dentist know; antibiotics can eliminate the risk. As for exercise, most people with MVP can follow a sensible program. Ask your doctor for guidance.

WARMING COLD HANDS

Q. *What causes cold hands, and what can I do about it?*

A. The most common cause, other than cold weather, is simple nervousness. When you're nervous, the surface capillaries in the hands and feet constrict, causing a feeling of coldness usually accompanied by localized sweating.

Less commonly, cold hands can reflect Raynaud's syndrome. When exposed to cold, the fingers or toes actually turn white. This change is caused by spasm of the arteries that supply them (without sweating). Drugs such as nifedipine (*Procardia*) and prazosin (*Minipress*), available by prescription, can help. Occasionally, biofeedback techniques are useful.

WALK AWAY FROM LEG PAIN

Q. *I suffer from leg pain because of poor circulation. Consumer Reports on Health mentioned that it's possible to relieve the condition by exercising. What type of exercise do you suggest?*

A. Simply walking, typically for a total of a half hour to an hour per day. The most effective regimen involves walking to the point of pain, stopping and waiting for the pain to subside, and then starting up again. But check with your physician first to make sure that would be safe for you.

ESOPHAGEAL SPASM

Q. *How can you tell chest pain caused by angina from that caused by a spasm of the esophagus?*

A. It's not always easy. Both types of pain are typically felt behind the breastbone. And the pain caused by an esophageal spasm often responds to nitroglycerin, the heart medication used to treat angina. However, there are three characteristics that do tend to set esophageal pain apart: (1) Unlike angina, it's more likely to occur when you're at rest; (2) it's often related to eating; and (3) it may be accompanied by difficulty in swallowing.

Since it can be difficult to tell the two disorders apart by symptoms alone, your physician may need to do some specific testing. Angina is usually evaluated by an exercise test (usually a treadmill test); esophageal spasm can be determined by a manometric test, in which you swallow a tube that measures esophageal muscle tension.

✚ Office Visit

CHEST PAIN: THE HEART OF THE MATTER

The pain in my chest intensifies as I reach for a book on the shelf behind my desk. Inevitably, the fear of heart attack accompanies any chest pain. But I remember last night's squash match and the lunge to make a point. The pain dulls as I drop my arm and returns when I lift it again. Making that shot apparently cost me a strained chest muscle.

Chest pain often has nothing to do with coronary disease. Most of my patients with chest pain have no cardiovascular problem at all. The cause of the chest pain is usually some minor, temporary problem—like my squash injury. In some cases, a serious chronic condition other than coronary disease is responsible for chest pain.

WHERE DOES IT HURT?

Patients who come to me with chest pain often have minor musculoskeletal problems. Unlike cardiac pain, pain from a strained chest muscle intensifies and subsides as the strained muscle fibers contract and relax when you move. This pain can last for days.

An injury to your ribs or breastbone can cause severe chest pain. You can usually identify such contusions and fractures because they're tender to the touch. Pain from a fractured rib can last for weeks. (Occasionally, arthritis affects one or more joints between the ribs and breastbone, causing chest pain.)

One of the most common sources of chest-pain complaints is heartburn, a burning sensation beneath your breastbone that worsens when you lie down. Typically, stomach acid flows up into the lower part of the esophagus, resulting in painful inflammation of the esophageal lining. That reflux may be caused by a hiatal hernia (when a part of the stomach protrudes through the diaphragm) or by overindulgence at the dinner table.

Some people have chest pain as a result of muscle spasms in the esophagus. Spasms typically occur during or shortly after meals, causing painful pressure in the center of the chest. Swallowing becomes difficult, and saliva accumulates in the mouth. Despite these distinguishing features, pain from esophageal spasms is often mistaken for a symptom of coronary disease. The masquerade is made more convincing because the pain may be relieved by drugs often prescribed for cardiac pain.

If the chest pain is sharp and increases with breathing, the problem is likely to be pleurisy, which is an inflammation of the lining of the lungs often caused by pneumonia or a pulmonary embolism (blood clot to the lung). That pain is sometimes accompanied by fever and shortness of breath, and prompt medical care is vital.

One disorder that's especially difficult to distinguish from true coronary disease is pericarditis, an inflammation of the heart lining. This condition occurs most often in young adults and is usually caused by a viral infection accompanied by aches, chills, and fever.

Problems in other organs—some too far from the heart to seem likely suspects—occasionally lead to chest pain. Disorders of the gallbladder and pancreas can cause pain in the lower chest and upper abdomen. Gallbladder inflammation also causes pain near the right shoulder blade; pancreatic problems can bring on intense discomfort in the midback.

Chest pain—often with heart "palpitations" and sweating—may be caused by emotional problems, especially severe anxiety and panic disorders.

WHEN PAIN COMES FROM THE HEART

Despite the wide range of possible causes of chest pain, nearly everyone thinks first of heart attack and coronary disease. The classic symptom of coronary disease is angina pectoris. Angina indicates that the heart muscle isn't getting enough oxygen because of decreased blood flow. Angina is typically a heavy, oppressive sensation in the center of the chest. The discomfort can radiate to the lower jaw, one or both arms (usually the left), and the upper back and neck. Angina generally strikes during physical exertion or emotional stress and can last as long as half an hour. More typically, the discomfort subsides within a few minutes when the exertion or stress ends.

Angina may be a precursor of a heart attack, which occurs when prolonged oxygen deprivation leads to the death of a portion of heart muscle. The pain of a heart attack resembles angina but typically lasts longer and is a more severe, crushing sensation. A heart attack is often accompanied by clammy skin, sweating, nausea, shortness of breath, and weakness.

If you've never had chest pain before and it strikes during physical exertion, call your physician immediately. If symptoms don't subside with rest, take an aspirin, and call 911 to transport you quickly to the nearest hospital emergency room. When a heart attack is coming on, every minute counts. Immediate treatment in the ambulance and at the hospital can be life-saving.

Children's health

STRENGTH TRAINING: SAFE FOR KIDS

Q. *I've always heard that muscle-building exercise will "stunt a child's growth." Now I hear it's recommended for children. Is strength training safe for kids?*

A. It won't inhibit growth under any circumstances, but it can cause injury—usually when lifting heavy weights with incorrect form. However, if it's carefully supervised and correctly done, strength training can actually reduce the risk of sports injuries in youngsters, since greater muscular strength and endurance help protect the joints and tendons. With proper safeguards, strength training can start whenever a child shows interest in the activity.

TONSIL TROUBLE

Q. My 9-year-old daughter has had swollen tonsils almost every month for the past two years. Our pediatrician repeatedly prescribes an antibiotic, which does help. I know tonsils no longer are removed routinely, but I wonder whether something more than a prescription is in order. Should I be so concerned?

A. Tonsillitis is usually caused by a strep infection and (when it's strep) is treated with antibiotics. Your daughter is a demonstration of how far the pendulum of medical opinion has swung away from the other treatment, tonsillectomy. Years ago there would have been no question. She would have been among the million people each year, most of them children, who had their tonsils removed. Today the number of operations is only about one-fourth as great; hers is a borderline case.

Surgery is certainly not necessary for your child, as long as her tonsils are not so swollen that they obstruct breathing or swallowing. Instead, the American Academy of Pediatrics says surgery is "a reasonable option" for a child who has many severe sore throats, especially if they are caused by strep.

How much will it help? For children with frequent sore throats, the operation has been shown to reduce the number of sore throats for a couple of years; after that the improvement appears to be slight. Considering the costs and risks, surgery might be indicated if she's now missing a significant amount of school.

WHICH MILK FOR KIDS?

Q. *What's the best milk for our 4-year-old? My wife says whole, the doctor says 2 percent, and I say 1 percent or skim milk. I contend that the difference in calories can be made up by offering more nutritious snacks.*

A. The only firm rules are for infants: The American Academy of Pediatrics recommends no cow's milk under age 1, and no reduced-fat milk under age 2. After children turn 2 and their need for fat diminishes, many pediatricians recommend switching to 1 percent or 2 percent milk. That's a good compromise between a child's need for a reliable, nutritious source of calories and the desire to instill a low-fat diet as a lifelong habit. However, doctors may modify their advice when a child is obese, is failing to thrive, or has an elevated risk of cardiovascular disease.

WHEN TO CHECK FOR STREP?

Q. *I'm sick and tired of hauling all three of my kids across town to the doctor every time they get sore throats, yet fear of untreated strep and its possible complications keeps me running to the doctor every time. Our family spent $250 in doctor visits this week. Are my concerns valid? And if so, can't my physician treat the family prophylactically without seeing each of us?*

A. Your concerns about strep are indeed valid. In a small minority of cases, untreated streptococcal infections can cause rheumatic fever or kidney disease. Treatment with antibiotics can prevent those complications. But only a throat culture can tell whether a sore throat is caused by strep and therefore requires antibiotic therapy.

Nevertheless, you may be able to lower your medical bills in some circumstances. If a child has sniffles and a cough as well as a sore throat, then it's unlikely to be strep; a phone call to the doctor may be all you need. On the other hand, if all three children are sick at the same time with sore throats, fever, and lymph-node enlargement—the typical signs of strep throat—and if one of them has a positive strep culture, then you can assume that the other two are probably also infected. In that case, all three can be treated with antibiotics simultaneously. (There is no reason for a doctor to give antibiotics prophylactically to family members who have no symptoms of strep.)

You might also ask your doctor whether he or she can take a throat culture without charging for a full office visit. Some doctors may be willing to do that if a full exam turns out to be unnecessary.

CONSTIPATED CHILD

Q. *For the past six months, our three-year-old son has averaged five days or more between bowel movements. We've tried to give him lots of natural fiber and fluids. On the advice of our pediatrician, we gave our son a stool softener for three weeks, but it hasn't helped. Should we keep using it?*

A. Prolonged use of a stool softener in children is not a good idea. Constipation in a 3-year-old is a common problem. In addition to lack of fiber or fluid in the diet, possible causes include resistance to toilet training, painful anal fissures, or even Hirschsprung's disease (a lack of muscle tone in part of the colon). Ask your pediatrician to refer you to a pediatric gastroenterologist, who may be better able to diagnose and treat the problem.

BED-WETTING

Q. *My 11-year-old daughter occasionally wets her bed. Why is this happening, and what can we do about it?*

A. In most cases, the cause of bed-wetting is unknown. However, psychological stress from such changes as the birth of a sibling or separation from a parent is often responsible. That's especially likely if the child has begun to wet the bed again a year or more after being successfully toilet trained. Rarely, bed-wetting is caused by an underlying disorder, such as diabetes, infection, or seizures.

Once a physical problem has been ruled out, handle bed-wetting with gentle measures. Avoid mechanical devices that use frightening alarms and electric shocks. Limit fluids after supper. Be sure your daughter urinates just before bedtime. Wake her up to urinate several hours after she's gone to sleep. Praise and reward her for a dry night; don't scold or punish for a wet night. If the problem persists, a brief course of the drug imipramine (*Tofranil*) can help a child gain control by helping to close the urethral sphincter, the muscle that stops the flow of urine. Even if all those measures fail, most children outgrow bed-wetting by adolescence.

Cholesterol

BETA-BLOCKERS AND CHOLESTEROL

Q. *Do the blood-pressure drugs known as beta-blockers affect cholesterol levels? I take* Lopressor *to control hypertension, and I'm concerned because I have a very high cholesterol level.*

A. While beta-blockers, including metoprolol *(Lopressor),* have been reported to raise triglycerides and lower levels of HDL (high-density lipoprotein, the "good" cholesterol), it is unclear how great the effects are and how they might affect the prognosis for coronary heart disease. These changes do not appear to affect total cholesterol or LDL (low-density lipoprotein, "bad" cholesterol) levels.

CHOLESTEROL AND COFFEE . . .

Q. *I've read that unfiltered brewed coffee can raise blood-cholesterol levels. But what about instant coffee? Can it raise cholesterol, too?*

A. Apparently not. That's because the manufacturing process removes nearly all of the two compounds—cafestol and kahweol—responsible for the increased cholesterol levels.

. . . AND DECAF

Q. *Does decaffeinated coffee contain the compounds that can raise cholesterol levels?*

A. That depends solely on how it's prepared. The decaffeination process itself has no effect on the offending substances —cafestol and kahweol. But like regular coffee, decaf that's instant or drip-filtered will have virtually none of those chemicals.

CHOLESTEROL-LOWERING DRUGS AND CATARACTS

Q. *My doctor wants to put me on medication to lower my cholesterol. But I read somewhere that the current cholesterol-lowering drugs can cause cataracts. Is that true?*

A. Only one cholesterol-lowering drug, lovastatin (*Mevacor*), was thought to have been associated with any risk of cataracts. And while that risk was believed to be quite low, the FDA advised users to get an annual exam for cataracts.

Yet several studies have now disproved any such association. The latest, a two-year study, found no difference between lovastatin and a placebo in forming cataracts. The annual examination for cataracts is no longer recommended for lovastatin users.

CONFUSION OVER HDL AND LDL

Q. *You seem to discuss HDL and LDL as if they were two types of cholesterol. But then you say that both HDL and LDL transport cholesterol. I'm confused.*

A. The terminology is confusing. HDL (high-density lipoprotein) and LDL (low-density lipoprotein) are not types of cholesterol. Rather, they're fat-protein compounds that transport cholesterol through the blood. (HDL tends to carry cholesterol away from the arteries, thus earning the title of "good" cholesterol; LDL, or "bad" cholesterol, tends to deposit cholesterol in the walls of arteries.)

When cholesterol is attached to a lipoprotein, the entire complex is properly referred to as HDL or LDL cholesterol. Sometimes, though, HDL and LDL are used as shorthand terms to refer to the lipoproteins together with their cholesterol cargo.

EATING BEFORE CHOLESTEROL TESTS

Q. *I had my cholesterol tested recently at a health fair. The previous day, I ate two meals with lots of fat and cholesterol. Did that throw off my cholesterol reading?*

A. No. Levels of total cholesterol don't change much from day to day. So you don't have to fast or worry about what you eat the day before a test. But if you were having blood drawn for a complete lipid analysis, including HDL cholesterol and triglycerides, then a 12- to 14-hour fast would be required.

THE GALLBLADDER AND CHOLESTEROL

Q. *My blood-cholesterol levels are high despite a low-fat diet. Could that have anything to do with the removal of my gallbladder 20 years ago?*

A. No. The gallbladder stores, concentrates, and regulates the flow of bile, which helps digest fats. But removing it has no noticeable effect on digestion and no effect at all on blood-cholesterol levels.

HDL FROM FOOD

Q. *We're constantly hearing about the opposing effects of high-density and low-density lipoprotein cholesterol in our blood, but when food is discussed, the distinction is dropped. Does the amount of HDL or LDL cholesterol in food affect the levels in our blood?*

A. No. Those lipoprotein-cholesterol combinations are broken down and reassembled within your body from their separate components—amino acids, cholesterol, and fats.

HIGH CHOLESTEROL, HIGH HDL

Q. *I'm a 64-year-old man with a total cholesterol level of 225, despite a very-low-fat diet. My HDL and triglyceride levels are both 67. Since my HDL level is high, my doctor says I don't need to take cholesterol-lowering drugs. Do you agree?*

A. Yes. Based on the numbers you provide, your level of LDL cholesterol (the "bad" kind) would be about 145, which is only mildly elevated and not in need of reduction by medication. And since your level of HDL cholesterol (the "good" kind) is so high (normal for men is 35 to 45), your risk of coronary heart disease due to cholesterol is relatively low.

HIGH CHOLESTEROL, LOW RISK

Q. *Last year, a lipoprotein analysis showed I had a total cholesterol level of 276 mg/dl, an LDL of 188 mg/dl, and an HDL of 77 mg/dl. My doctor says these results indicate a low risk of coronary heart disease. I eat a low-fat diet, I'm active, and my weight is good. Yet you have suggested that drug therapy may be necessary for such a high LDL level. Is it necessary for me?*

A. Probably not. As we said, before putting you on medication your physician should consider a number of variables, including your personal and family medical histories and any other risk factors for coronary disease. Based on your high level of HDL ("good") cholesterol and your health habits, it sounds as if your risk factors are indeed well under control.

JUMPING CHOLESTEROL

Q. *According to a finger-prick test, my blood-cholesterol level was 197. Two months later, it was 272 on a fasting blood workup. My diet didn't change during that time. Is such a jump possible in only two months?*

A. No. Cholesterol readings cannot vary that much, that soon. The finger-prick test was probably wrong. Squeezing the fingertip to draw blood produces secretions that dilute the blood and can lead to a falsely low reading.

NIACIN ALERT

Q. *I recently read that the sustained-release form of niacin, which I've been taking to control my blood cholesterol, can cause liver damage. Why is this form of niacin dangerous, but the regular crystalline form, which causes me to flush, is not?*

A. It's long been known that both crystalline (short-acting) and sustained-release niacin can damage the liver at high doses. It now seems that the sustained-release form can cause liver injury even at low therapeutic doses. In several case reports, people who had recovered from such damage were then given crystalline niacin, with no ill effects. The reason for the difference is unclear; it may be that taking short-acting crystalline niacin allows the liver to recover between dosages while slow-release niacin affects liver enzyme systems for longer durations and with fewer recovery periods.

Another report suggests that high doses of niacin can aggravate diabetes and may induce the disease in borderline diabetics. Although niacin is available without a prescription, it should nevertheless be taken under a doctor's supervision and only in crystalline form. Increasing the dosage very slowly to the target level will minimize any uncomfortable facial flushing.

LONG-TERM CHOLESTEROL MEDICATION

Q. *For two years, I've taken Lopid, which has lowered my cholesterol level from 280 to 230. My doctor wants me to keep taking it indefinitely. What are the long-term side effects?*

A. Gallstones, but they're rare. Even short-term side effects of gemfibrozil (*Lopid*) develop only infrequently; those can include digestive disturbances, impaired liver function, and muscle pains. If the drug hasn't caused side effects after two years, it probably never will.

Keep in mind, too, that if you decide to stop taking the drug, your cholesterol will probably shoot back up again.

SOARING CHOLESTEROL

Q. *My 57-year-old wife has a cholesterol level of 520 mg/dl. We eat the same foods, and my blood cholesterol is only 170 mg/dl. Her blood pressure is normal, she's not overweight, and she doesn't smoke, drink, or have diabetes. After four weeks on* Mevacor, *her cholesterol level dropped to 340 mg/dl. But she developed painfully swollen ankles and now refuses to take this or any other cholesterol-lowering drug. What do you recommend?*

A. Swollen ankles are not a known side effect of lovastatin (*Mevacor*). Your wife should get back on cholesterol-lowering medication and look for another possible cause of her swollen ankles.

A blood-cholesterol level of 520 mg/dl is uncommon and ominous. Such high cholesterol, usually an inherited disorder, often causes coronary heart disease at a relatively early age.

TRIGLYCERIDES AND DIET

Q. *What type of diet will lower triglyceride levels?*

A. The same low-fat diet that can lower blood-cholesterol levels often lowers triglyceride levels as well. Avoiding alcohol and, for some people, cutting back on carbohydrates can also reduce triglyceride levels.

. . . AND ESTROGEN

Q. *I'm a 65-year-old woman. My gynecologist wants me to take estrogen because the hormone would improve my cholesterol levels. But my internist warns that it would raise my triglyceride levels. What's the net effect?*

A. Overall, hormone replacement therapy helps protect women against coronary heart disease. That's apparently because estrogen tends to decrease LDL, the "bad" cholesterol, and increase HDL, the "good" kind. It's possible that estrogen use might be even more protective if it didn't also raise triglycerides in some women. But for most women, the hormone's positive effect on cholesterol outweighs its negative effect on triglyceride levels.

Colon and rectal complaints

ANAL ITCHING

Q. *I have been suffering from severe pruritus ani for nearly a year. To find relief from the itching, I've been to a family physician, a proctologist, four dermatologists, and an allergist. So far, no treatment has helped. Do you know of anything that might relieve my discomfort?*

A. Since you've already seen seven doctors, they've probably ruled out the most common causes of anal itching: worms, hemorrhoids, fungal infections, skin fissures, sweating, irritants in food, and poor anal hygiene.

One possibility that's sometimes overlooked is neurodermatitis. This is not an actual nerve disorder but rather a lengthy cycle of itching and repeated scratching. It leads to gradual thickening of the skin around the anus, which then itches more than ever.

If neurodermatitis is indeed the cause of your condition, it may gradually abate if you force yourself not to scratch the thickened skin. When you're at home, applying an ice-cold compress to the irritated area can ease the urge to scratch. Since many sufferers scratch when they're asleep, you should keep your fingernails short and even wear soft mittens to bed. A hypnotist or psychotherapist might help you stop scratching.

ANAL FISSURES

Q. *I've been taking a tablespoon of mineral oil every night for many years to prevent anal fissures. Is this bad for me?*

A. Yes. Mineral oil decreases absorption of fat-soluble vitamins (A, D, E, and K), and can cause an unusual type of pneumonia if inhaled. Try a stool softener (*Dialose, Pro-Cal-Sof*) or psyllium laxative (*Metamucil, Mylanta Natural Fiber*) to minimize trauma to the anal area during bowel movements. A warm bath for 10 to 15 minutes after bowel movements may bring some relief. Fissures that persist may require surgery.

BLOOD IN THE STOOL

Q. *Microscopic traces of blood have been detected in my stool. Sigmoidoscopy revealed internal hemorrhoids near the entrance of the anus. Does this mean surgery, even though I've had no discomfort?*

A. Not necessarily. Stool softeners (*Dialose, Pro-Cal-Sof*) or psyllium laxatives (*Metamucil, Mylanta Natural Fiber*) can reduce straining during bowel movements and may help stop the bleeding, just as they help prevent anal fissures. Antihemorrhoidal creams and suppositories are not particularly helpful for this problem. Like persistent fissures, persistent bleeding may require surgery.

COLONOSCOPY PAIN

Q. *Because of a strong family history of colon cancer, doctors have advised me to have an annual colonoscopy. I've undergone the procedure a few times and found the pain nearly unbearable. My gastroenterologist says he doesn't give painkillers for colonoscopy. Is there anything that would help me cope with this ordeal?*

A. Yes—drugs, including those painkillers. Without them, the colonoscope causes discomfort and sometimes pain as it snakes through and stretches your colon. Before the procedure, most gastroenterologists give intravenous narcotics to kill pain and tranquilizers to relax the colon. If you can't persuade your gastroenterologist to administer such medications, try another gastroenterologist.

DIET AND DIVERTICULOSIS

Q. *Like many people my age (over 50), I have diverticulosis. My doctor has told me not to eat seeds and nuts and to avoid constipation. But I know people with the same problem who have been told to eat, avoid, or do different things. Could you provide some insight into this problem?*

A. Diverticulosis is a common condition in which the inner lining of the intestine protrudes through the intestinal wall, forming small sacs or pouches in the colon. It affects one in four people by the age of 50 and is near-universal by the age of 80. It's believed that our modern low-fiber diet is at least partly to blame.

Diverticulosis usually doesn't cause any symptoms, but some people with the condition do experience bloating, cramps, and changed bowel habits, such as constipation, diarrhea, or alternating attacks of both. Abdominal pain (especially low on the left side) accompanied by fever might signal the development of diverticulitis, an infection of the sacs. That can lead to abscess formation and to perforation of the bowel, which can cause peritonitis, a generalized infection of the abdominal lining.

To avoid those problems, switch gradually to a higher-fiber diet with more whole grains, fruits, and vegetables. Avoid seeds and nuts; small and hard to digest, they can get trapped in the tiny pouches and may cause inflammation.

ULCERATIVE COLITIS

Q. *I recently found out I have ulcerative colitis. What's the latest on the cause and treatment of this disease?*

A. Physicians still don't know what causes ulcerative colitis, an inflammatory disease of the colon that leads to diarrhea and rectal bleeding. (It can also affect the skin, eyes, joints, and liver.) However, various drugs can suppress the inflammation and control the symptoms. Those medications include mesalamine (*Asacol*) and sulfasalazine (*Azulfidine*), corticosteroid drugs such as prednisone (*Deltasone*), and in resistant cases, immunosuppressant drugs such as mercaptopurine (*Purinethol*).

People who have had extensive ulcerative colitis for a long time may be at increased risk of colon cancer. Those people should undergo periodic colonoscopy (inspection of the entire colon through a flexible lighted tube) to check for cancer or precancerous changes.

Cysts, lumps, and tumors

BENIGN CHANGES IN THE BREAST

Q. *Six months ago I had a breast biopsy that showed benign changes—fibrocystic disease and intraductal hyperplasia. Is either of these linked to an increased risk of breast cancer in the absence of a family history?*

A. Your risk of breast cancer is no greater than average. The conditions you mention are natural changes that occur over time. Fibrocystic "disease," a term that implies an abnormality or disorder, is a misnomer, since about half of all premenopausal women have it. It's really a catchall term for painful, lumpy breasts. Such lumps were once thought to be associated with increased cancer risk, but several studies have since dispelled that notion. Intraductal hyperplasia is a benign overgrowth of cells in the breast ducts, the tubes that carry milk to the nipple. Only when those cells start to appear abnormal on a biopsy does the risk of cancer increase.

BREAST LUMPS

Q. *At the time of my last routine physical, my doctor diagnosed a fibrocystic lump in my breast. I was told to avoid anything containing caffeine, including chocolate. But I love chocolate. Would eating chocolate really affect the growth of any lumps?*

A. Probably not. The theory that caffeine causes noncancerous breast lumps has never been proved. Besides, chocolate contains relatively small amounts of caffeine.

FIBROID TUMORS AND ESTROGEN

Q. *For years my doctor told me that I could never go on estrogen replacement therapy because I have a fibroid tumor on my uterus (roughly the size of a 14-week fetus). I've just reached menopause, and now he's changed his mind; he wants me to start hormone therapy. He says it would be okay—that the tumor would even shrink. Please advise.*

A. Estrogen can stimulate the growth of uterine fibroids, which are benign tumors of muscle and connective tissue that originate within the uterine wall. Now that you have reached menopause, your body's own supply of the hormone has begun to dwindle. Ordinarily, that would make the tumor shrink. The tumor might continue to shrink even with estrogen replacement therapy, if the dose of estrogen was relatively low. Higher doses might maintain the tumor or even make it grow.

If you decide to go on estrogen replacement therapy—because of severe menopausal symptoms, for example, or a high risk of osteoporosis or coronary heart disease—your fibroid tumor should be monitored closely. If it continues to grow, your physician may reduce your estrogen dosage or suggest that you stop taking the hormone entirely.

BODY BUMPS

Q. *I have several egg-shaped growths on my body. Please explain whether these bumps, diagnosed as lipomas, are dangerous and how the condition can be treated. I would have quite a few scars if the lumps were all surgically removed.*

A. Lipomas are benign, fatty tumors that are fairly common, typically appearing on the trunk, neck, and forearms. Usually they cause no discomfort and are best left alone. If you prefer to have them removed for cosmetic reasons, you can choose either conventional surgery or liposuction, in which a small tube inserted under the skin sucks out the fatty tissue, resulting in less scar formation. The rare lipoma that enlarges rapidly may harbor a cancerous growth, known as a liposarcoma, and should be removed surgically.

Dental care

DENTAL X-RAYS

Q. *I'm 40 years old and haven't had a cavity since I was 10. Yet my dentist recommends annual X-rays to look between the back teeth for cavities. Doesn't this expose me to too much radiation?*

A. Overall, the risk from dental X-rays is minimal. Today, a full-mouth series of X-rays exposes patients to only 13 millirems of radiation. By comparison, Americans are exposed to 300 millirems a year just from the natural environment. But if you have no history of cavities and your gums are healthy, too, there's little reason for annual X-rays. Talk to your dentist about having "bitewing" X-rays every two or three years, instead; they target the specific teeth the dentist is concerned about.

ALTERNATIVES TO TOOTH CAPS

Q. *I have a gap between my two front teeth. Dentists have previously advised against grinding down two or four otherwise healthy teeth to cap them. Can anything else be done?*

A. There are newer procedures for improving the appearance of your teeth without cutting them down or covering them with caps. Teeth can be reshaped, and spaces closed, by bonding with composites, porcelain, or plastic veneers. Ask your dentist about the relative cost and durability of the various procedures.

BRACES: HEALTH OR BEAUTY?

Q. *Most children in my son's class have braces on their teeth, and our orthodontist is suggesting we have our son fitted, too. Are there good medical and dental reasons for giving children perfectly straight teeth, or is the main motivation cosmetic?*

A. It's mostly cosmetic. Crooked teeth can certainly cause emotional distress, particularly in appearance-conscious teens. But the reasons usually given for straightening a child's teeth—to prevent cavities and gum disease—have been questioned after a number of studies failed to show a protective effect. Nor have researchers convincingly linked crooked teeth to temporomandibular joint (TMJ) syndrome. Only a severely disordered bite is likely to cause such physical problems as difficulty chewing or gum disease.

CALCIUM FOR ORAL HEALTH?

Q. *I'm a 42-year-old woman with receding gums and bone loss around my teeth. My dentist recommends that I take calcium supplements to delay further bone loss. Is this the best treatment for my condition?*

A. There's no evidence that getting extra calcium will help reduce periodontal disease, which is what causes such bone loss. You should be evaluated by a periodontist. Treatment options range from periodic root planing to various surgical therapies.

CAN RECEDING GUMS BE REBUILT?

Q. *I am almost 60 years old and have near-perfect teeth. But my gums are receding. I recall reading about an innovative technique in which a gumlike substance is attached to the teeth along the receding gum line. Can you tell me more about this approach?*

A. The technique you read about may have been guided tissue regeneration. A porous membrane placed between the gum and the tooth encourages connective tissue to cross the membrane and bind to the root. The technique helps close periodontal pockets, the spaces between gums and roots where infection breeds. But such a procedure doesn't grow new gum tissue to cover the exposed roots.

DENTAL PLANING VS. CLEANING

Q. *For some years I've had my teeth cleaned twice a year, at a cost of $25 to $35 per visit. A new dentist recently recommended that I have dental planing done. But the cost for planing is $120 a visit, and each visit deals with only one-quarter of my teeth. Please comment.*

A. There's a big difference between cleaning and planing, in function as well as cost. Cleaning removes tartar above and around the gum line and polishes the teeth. It's often performed by a dental hygienist. Planing, on the other hand, may be necessary to prevent the progression of gum disease. The procedure removes hard and soft deposits on root surfaces beneath the gum line and smoothes, or planes, root surfaces. It's often performed under local anesthesia or nitrous oxide, and only by a dentist. For that reason, it costs much more than ordinary cleaning.

DENTAL X-RAYS

Q. *How often should I have dental X-rays? My dentist says every six months is safe, but that strikes me as excessive—and expensive.*

A. If you're prone to tooth decay, you might need bitewing X-rays as often as every six months. However, most people with healthy teeth can go one or two years between such X-rays. Full-mouth X-rays are generally needed much less often—about once every five years—to assess the overall health of the teeth and supporting tissue in adults. Modern X-ray equipment, as well as a lead apron and collar shield, minimizes the radiation exposure.

FILLINGS AND PINS

Q. *When filling cavities in my teeth, my dentist installed pins to hold the fillings in place. Is this a new procedure, and is it really helpful?*

A. That practice has been around for quite some time. It's helpful when you've lost a good part of the tooth structure. The dentist threads pins into the tooth's dentin (the layer under the enamel) to serve as a support for the filling.

FLUORIDE SUPPLEMENTS

Q. *Are sodium fluoride supplements safe for my two-year-old child?*

A. Yes, in the correct dosage. Fluoride supplements (drops or tablets) may be prescribed for children when the fluoride content of local drinking water is less than 0.3 parts per million. The recommended daily dosage is 0.25 milligram up to the age of two, 0.5 milligram from age two to three, and 1 milligram from age three to age 14, when the second molars have usually erupted fully. After that, fluoride from toothpaste and fluoride treatments at the dentist's office provide sufficient protection.

Some years ago, when the recommended dosage for children up to age two was higher (0.5 milligram), there was some concern about mild dental fluorosis—faint white spots on the teeth. But that minor side effect rarely occurs today.

IMPLANT OR BRIDGE?

Q. *I have a lower molar that needs to be replaced soon. My dentist has suggested a bridge, and said that bridges have been proved to be reliable. I'm interested in a more modern technique—getting a false tooth supported by a pole implanted in the jawbone. How much research has been done on that?*

A. Implants have an advantage over bridges, in that they don't damage adjacent teeth. To install a bridge, the dentist must first file down the adjacent teeth and then crown them. Single-tooth implants have most often been used to replace upper front teeth, a procedure that is usually successful. However, the value of implants in replacing single back teeth has been less thoroughly studied. An implant can be used only if there is enough bone left under the gum to anchor it, and only in locations where the implanting procedure could not damage a nerve or sinus cavity. A dentist performing implants should have gone through a formal educational program in implant techniques.

The cost of implants and bridges is roughly comparable—generally around $3,000 for a single-tooth implant and a few hundred dollars less for a bridge. But some insurers that cover bridges do not cover implants.

PERIODONTAL SURGERY

Q. *My periodontist wants to trim back the gums around six of my teeth, although he says it's a gamble whether that will stabilize my periodontal disease. Friends have told me to save my money ($600 to $700) because it didn't work for them. Should I have the surgery?*

A. You can't predict the outcome of gum surgery from your friends' experiences. But you should consider surgery only after other measures have failed to stop the progression of the disease. Those measures include a combination of instructed self-care (brushing, flossing, dental rinse) and professional scaling and root planing. It would be wise to get a second opinion before you decide on surgery.

SACCHARIN SMILE

Q. *After years of being told to avoid saccharin, I see it's in many toothpastes. Is it safe?*

A. Yes. The amount you'd ingest from toothpaste is insignificant.

TARTAR CONTROL

Q. *My dental hygienist told me that I have an unusually heavy buildup of tartar. Since I already floss nightly, she suggested that I try either an antiseptic mouthwash such as* Listerine *or a toothpaste containing baking soda, or else start flossing twice a day. What should I do?*

A. There's no need to floss twice a day, but be sure to use the proper technique when you do floss: Don't just work the thread between teeth with a sawing motion; curve it around each tooth and sweep it up and down across the broad surfaces.

Since you seem to develop tartar especially quickly, try brushing twice a day with a tartar-control toothpaste. (If you develop a rash around the outside of your mouth, try switching brands.) You should also continue to get periodic professional cleanings.

Listerine can fight plaque, but it doesn't slow the conversion of plaque to tartar. Toothpastes containing baking soda, or bicarbonate, may actually encourage tartar formation, at least theoretically, by increasing the alkalinity of the mouth.

TIME FOR A CROWN?

Q. *At my last checkup, my dentist told me that large silver fillings in two molars were deteriorating and that crowns would be necessary. Couldn't I just have the fillings replaced?*

A. Possibly, but that may not be the best solution. The average filling starts deteriorating after about 10 years. When you need a replacement, the tooth must be hollowed out further to accommodate the new filling. But if the old filling is large to begin with, removing more of the tooth could make it vulnerable to fracture from chewing. Often, the wiser choice may be a crown, which is more expensive than a filling but lasts much longer. The tooth is first filed down, and a crown made of porcelain, gold, or plastic is then anchored to the stub.

TOOTHPICKS AND GUM DISEASE

Q. *I thought brushing and flossing were enough to prevent gingivitis. But my dentist says I should also use a toothpick. Is that necessary?*

A. Brushing and flossing are usually enough for most people. However, a pick can help if your gums are still inflamed or if they bleed during cleanings, both signs of early gum disease. You can use a regular toothpick or a commercial "interdental stimulator," such as *Stim-U-Dent.*

Once a day, massage your gums by moving the pick in and out of the spaces between your teeth several times. Your gums may bleed at first, but after a few days the swollen tissues repair themselves to a healthier condition. If bleeding persists, see your dentist.

TOOTH-DECAY DEFENSE

Q. *My children, ages 14 and 15, have no dental problems, but were recently advised by a new dentist to have their molars and premolars treated with sealants. What are the appropriate indications for this procedure?*

A. Sealants are an excellent way to protect children's first and second permanent molars, even in the absence of current dental problems. The procedure involves applying a soft plastic to the tooth surface to fill in the pits and fissures. This prevents food and bacteria from accumulating in those spaces. The plastic is then hardened with a special light or chemical.

Sealants should be applied soon after the molars appear: at about age six to seven for the first molar, and age 12 to 14 for the second. Children with evidence of tooth decay may also benefit from sealants on their premolars, also called bicuspids, which appear at age 9 to 12.

WISDOM-TOOTH REMOVAL

Q. *After a series of X-rays, my dentist recommended removing my 13-year-old son's upper wisdom teeth at 15 for proper spacing. How seriously should I take this advice?*

A. This advice stems from the concern that impacted wisdom teeth, or third molars, will tend to push other teeth inward. But long-term studies have now shown that teeth can crowd together whether or not the wisdom teeth have been removed. Crowding, when it occurs, seems to result from a natural tendency of the teeth to move forward, although the exact causes are not clear.

Wisdom teeth should be removed when there is a better reason to do so, such as a painful infection around the teeth. Teeth that are merely impacted will not necessarily become troublesome over time. In addition, teeth that appear to be impacted at age 15 may right themselves in another five or six years. Since wisdom teeth generally don't reach their final position until the early twenties, it's too early to tell how your son's teeth will grow in.

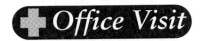

WITH IRWIN D. MANDEL, D.D.S.

BAD BREATH: WHAT YOUR BEST FRIEND CAN'T TELL YOU

Are you reluctant to open your mouth when your dentist or dental hygienist approaches? Many times, I've encountered patients who are—and not because they're afraid I'll hurt them. Rather, they're afraid they'll "offend."

Such fears are no doubt fueled by the inescapable ads for breath mints, sprays, washes, and pills. Surveys show that 55 to 75 million Americans now consider bad breath a principal concern in social encounters. But while chronic halitosis, the medical name for true bad breath, is not entirely a Madison Avenue myth, it's much less common than the ads or surveys suggest. When it is present, it's almost always due to problems in the mouth that can be readily remedied.

NATURAL BREATH ODORS

Certain breath odors are common, but they're generally mild and temporary. Many foods can taint your breath immediately after a meal. Two of the main offenders, garlic and onion, can actually stay on your breath for 24 hours or more. That's because the active chemical travels through the digestive system to the blood, to the lungs, and back out through the mouth. Even when rubbed on the skin, the odor of garlic eventually finds its way to the breath. Smoking and drinking, of course, also leave their distinctive mark on the breath.

If eating and drinking too much of some things are bad for your breath, eating too little can at times be no better. Dieters may develop the mildly unpleasant "hunger breath" when certain metabolic wastes reach the lungs. (A well-timed snack curbs hunger breath, but at some cost to the diet, of course.)

Then there's "morning breath." While you sleep, your tongue moves less and secretion of saliva slows almost to a standstill. Dead cells that are continually shed from the tissues lining your mouth are no longer rubbed off, washed away, and swallowed. The normal bacteria in the mouth break down those dead cells, releasing malodorous by-products. But the odor disappears as soon as you brush and floss your teeth, or even when you have something to eat or drink.

ORAL CARE AND ODOR CULPRITS

Problems involving the teeth, gums, and tongue are the main cause of true halitosis. Without scrupulous oral hygiene, the teeth become coated with bacterial plaque, which can eventually give rise to gum disease as well as tooth decay. And badly decayed teeth smell pretty bad. But even relatively mild gum disease can generate unpleasant odors, as plaque and its hardened form, tartar, create pockets that collect pus. For that matter, rotting food that's impacted around faulty fillings or just between the teeth can also create a stink.

Recent research shows that heavy bacterial plaques can also form on the back of the tongue. Because of its large, rough surface area, the tongue readily retains the bacteria, along with shed cells and even food debris. And the tongue bacteria are mostly the type that can easily putrefy those accumulations, generating a variety of sulfur compounds and other odoriferous substances.

If gum disease threatens your teeth and fouls your breath, you should seek professional care. But you can help prevent gum disease by keeping your mouth clean. That means brushing twice a day, flossing once, and getting regular professional cleanings.

You can also keep your tongue clean by brushing it gently once a day with a soft wet brush after you brush your teeth, or by periodically scraping the rear portion with a bent spoon. (You can even buy a specially designed tongue-scraper in a drugstore.)

If those measures are inadequate, you can add a potent mouthwash. So far, two types of products have substantial scientific evidence to back them up: *Listerine* and a prescription rinse available as *Peridex* and *PerioGard*. At least one small clinical trial suggests that mouth rinses containing the germicide chlorine dioxide—including *Oxyfresh, Closys II,* and other products, often sold directly by dentists—may also be helpful.

The widely advertised product *BreathAsure*—capsules containing parsley-seed and sunflower oils—built its success on claims that it eliminates bad breath by working within the digestive system. That's doubtful.

IF NOT DENTAL, MAYBE MEDICAL

If there's nothing wrong in your mouth, you may be one of the few people whose halitosis actually signals a medical problem. Most often, it's a local infection of the respiratory tract (the nose, throat, windpipe, and lungs), such as chronic sinusitis or bronchitis. Other possible medical causes include diabetes, kidney and liver disease, gastrointestinal problems, and rare metabolic disorders. Finally, halitosis can also result from anything that dries the mouth—fever, medications, salivary-gland disorders, or just breathing through your mouth.

But don't let all this give you the wrong impression. Bad breath requiring the attention of a dentist or physician is relatively uncommon. There's even evidence suggesting that as many as one in four people who believe they have chronic bad breath actually suffer from halitosis phobia. They'll often remain convinced of their offense despite objective evidence to the contrary.

Still, if you're concerned about your breath, ask a professional for an honest appraisal. Your best friend may not tell you, as the old commercial warned, but your dentist or doctor will.

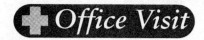

WITH IRWIN D. MANDEL, D.D.S.

EXAMINING YOUR DENTIST . . . AND FINDING A NEW ONE

The only thing worse than not seeing a dentist at all is seeing a bad one. Either way, you stand to lose your teeth. And if you stick with an inferior dentist, you'll lose your money as well.

Yet many people stay put when they should walk. Most of them probably don't even realize they're being inadequately treated, since that's not always obvious. To evaluate the kind of care you're getting, you'll have to ask yourself some probing questions. See if your dentist passes this dental exam:

DRILLING AND FILLING
Is your dentist a talented technician?
Patients can't judge a dentist's technical skills precisely. But you can usually distinguish good dentistry from bad.

During prolonged probing or drilling, a good dentist will occasionally pause so you can relax and rest your jaw. After any sort of dental work, your bite should feel natural and your gums should not bleed. Fillings shouldn't catch your tongue, interfere with flossing, or give food particles and plaque a toehold.

If the dentist does the job well, a silver filling should last at least 10 years, depending on its size and location; crowns and bridges generally last even longer.

Does your dentist minimize temporary measures?

Be wary if your dentist puts in one temporary filling after another instead of proceeding directly to a permanent filling. This may mean the dentist has a high-volume practice and isn't willing to spend enough time with you. Or it may simply mean more visits, and thus more fees.

TREATMENT AND OVERTREATMENT

Does your dentist discuss options?

Alternative treatments are more common in dentistry than in medicine. For example, a dentist may treat a tooth that has an especially deep cavity by doing root-canal work and then installing a silver filling; by inserting a gold inlay; by constructing a post and crown; or even by extracting the tooth. A good dentist should recommend the minimum treatment required to maintain dental health. When there are reasonable alternatives, your dentist should explain the pros and cons and let you decide.

Does your dentist respect your limits?

Tolerance for pain differs from person to person. If you can't bear the pain of dental work, your dentist should be willing to give you an adequate anesthetic or a sedative.

Does your dentist estimate and itemize?

Don't hesitate to ask for a written estimate of how long a

proposed treatment will take and how much it will cost. After treatment, you should get an itemized bill.

Does your dentist avoid unnecessary work?

Certain shady practices can alert you to an overzealous dentist. Take your business elsewhere if your dentist:

• Suggests replacing any silver amalgam fillings to protect you from the minute amount of mercury vapors they release when you chew. Overwhelming evidence supports the safety of amalgam fillings.

• Wants to cut down several teeth and install crowns. (While that can be necessary in extreme cases, you should at least get a second opinion.)

• Worries you about your appearance in order to sell you on some cosmetic dental procedure. (I'm all for cosmetic dentistry, but only if the motivation comes from the patient, not from the dentist.)

PREVENTING TROUBLE

Is your dentist prevention-minded?

This preventive approach should be apparent from the very first visit, when the dentist takes a thorough medical and dental history. Your dentist should also perform a complete "head and neck" examination at the initial visit and every few years thereafter. Such an exam should include inspection of your teeth, gums, jaw joint, facial muscles, and the inside of your mouth.

Does your dentist make you a partner in prevention?

Either the dentist or the dental hygienist should instruct you on how to care for your teeth. He or she should give you a refresher course from time to time, perhaps having you demonstrate your brushing and flossing techniques and suggesting improvements.

The dentist or hygienist should also advise you on such preventive extras as fluoride use, antibacterial rinses, and any supplemental oral hygiene aids you may need: an irrigator, a power brush, or floss threaders to clean around dental work.

Does your dentist invite you back?

A well-functioning recall system guarantees that no problem will go too far awry. In most cases, a checkup should be scheduled every six months to a year. At that time, the hygienist scales hardened plaque off your teeth and then polishes them. Unless something seems wrong, your dentist may not need to do much more than see that the hygienist has done a good job.

Does your dentist order X-rays responsibly?

With most patients, there's no reason to take a full series of X-rays more often than once every five years or so. A survey of decay with two to four X-rays, called bitewings, may be taken every year or two, depending on your susceptibility to decay. If a problem arises, of course, X-rays of the suspect area can be taken as needed. A dentist who never X-rays your teeth is just as bad as one who does it too often.

Does your dentist guard against infection?

Your dentist and hygienist should wear rubber gloves and a mask when treating you. Beyond that, your dentist should be willing to explain the other sanitation procedures used to protect patients and staff from infectious diseases.

HOW TO FIND A NEW DENTIST

If your dentist fails your examination—or if you're moving or you don't have a regular dentist—you'll need to find a new one. Don't turn to the Yellow Pages or local dental societies; they list dentists but don't evaluate them. Instead, try these sources:

• If there's a dental school nearby, call and ask for the names of practicing faculty members.

• If a hospital or health center provides dental services in your area, ask the dentist in charge for recommendations.

• If you already know an orthodontist or periodontist, ask

for the name of a good general practitioner. Those dental specialists should be familiar with the quality of work done by referring dentists.

• If you're moving and your current dentist meets most of the criteria I've discussed, ask whether he or she can recommend colleagues in your new location.

When you visit a dental office for the first time, the dentist and staff should be willing to answer all of your questions. If they're not, that's one sign that you ought to look elsewhere.

Diabetes

DIABETES AND BLOOD SUGAR

Q. *I'm a 42-year-old man, and my fasting blood sugar level is about 115-125 mg/dl. I have no family history of diabetes, am not overweight, and have had normal results on glucose-tolerance tests. But I'm afraid I may develop diabetes if my blood-sugar level stays high. How can I lower it?*

A. Other than stopping any medications (such as corticosteroids or thiazide diuretics) that might be boosting your blood sugar, there's really no way to lower your sugar level.

The American Diabetes Association has lowered the threshold for diagnosing diabetes to a fasting blood-sugar level of 126 mg/dl; a normal level can range up to 110 mg/dl. So your fasting blood-sugar level would be considered somewhat elevated. Aside from keeping your weight under control and getting regular exercise, the most important thing you should do is get tested for the disease at least every three years.

DIABETES DRUGS RISKY?

Q. *My doctor insists that I take* DiaBeta *twice a day. But I have read that oral antidiabetic medications boost the risk of heart disease. What should I do?*

A. Take the medication. That old warning was based on a single, seriously flawed study conducted more than 25 years ago. Untreated, diabetes results in persistently elevated blood-sugar levels, which can damage the eyes, heart, kidneys, and nerves. Those complications pose a much graver danger than any possible harm from the medication itself.

ASPIRIN AND DIABETICS

Q. *Is it true that aspirin can lower blood-sugar levels in diabetics?*

A. Yes, but only with prolonged use and in large amounts (eight or more 325-mg tablets a day). That reduction in blood-sugar levels can magnify the sugar-lowering effects of insulin and oral antidiabetic drugs. While such use of aspirin is generally safe for people with diabetes, they must be monitored closely by a physician.

Diet and nutrition

NO MEAT WITH POTATOES?

Q. *I've heard that you shouldn't combine foods that contain protein with foods that contain carbohydrates at one meal. Is there any sound basis for such advice?*

A. None whatsoever. After all, even individual foods are in themselves combinations of protein and carbohydrates, as well as fat.

ELEVATED POTASSIUM

Q. *Blood tests show that my potassium levels are higher than the maximum normal level of 5.5 millimoles per liter. I follow good health habits, including a careful diet. What could be causing that elevation?*

A. By far the most common reason is simply a faulty testing technique that churns the blood while drawing or analyzing it. This in turn releases potassium from the blood cells. However, the elevation might also be caused by potassium supplements, medications (such as certain diuretics, beta-blockers, or ACE inhibitors), kidney failure, insufficient secretion of adrenal hormones, or any one of several uncommon inherited diseases.

If repeated blood tests confirm that your potassium level is indeed above normal, you should be evaluated to find out what's wrong. Any further rise can be dangerous.

FROZEN BACTERIA

Q. *Does freezing destroy bacteria in food?*

A. No. Although growth stops and the total bacterial count may decline during freezing, plenty of microbes will survive. If frozen foods aren't safe before freezing, they won't be safe after thawing. Heat is the surest way to kill bacteria. The temperature and cooking time depend on the food.

FROZEN VEGETABLES

Q. *You've reported that frozen vegetables are often more nutritious than the fresh ones sold in supermarkets. And you said not to thaw them before cooking, so they'll retain nutrients. But how can I be sure frozen vegetables haven't thawed and refrozen at some point before I buy them?*

A. Feel the bag to make sure the vegetables aren't clumped together. If the bag is clear, check to see that there's no sign of ice crystallization inside. Boxed vegetables, of course, are forced into clumps, so it's harder to tell if they've thawed and refrozen. All you can do is avoid boxes with lots of ice crystals on them.

HONEY VS. SUGAR

Q. *Is honey nutritionally superior to plain table sugar?*

A. Not at all. In fact, honey and table sugar are nearly indistinguishable chemically; once digested, they're identical. Neither sweetener has any nutritional value other than calories.

Teaspoon for teaspoon, however, table sugar actually contains fewer calories than honey (16 vs. 22). That's because the dry crystals take up more space than the dissolved sugars of honey.

LACTOSE INTOLERANCE

Q. *What diet should a person with lactose intolerance follow?*

A. Without the enzyme lactase, the body is unable to break down milk sugar (lactose) into simple sugars that can be absorbed. People deficient in this enzyme can't completely digest milk and milk products, especially cheese and ice cream. Small amounts of those foods usually cause no problem, but too much can result in cramps, bloating, diarrhea, and flatulence.

If you're highly intolerant to lactose, you can take lactase capsules or tablets (*Dairy Ease, LactAid, Lactrase*) before you ingest milk products. *LactAid* is also available as a liquid concentrate that you add to regular milk. And lactose-reduced milk (also sold under the brand name *LactAid*) is available in food stores.

PICK-ME-UP PILL

Q. *Five years ago I began taking one tablet of* Vivarin *each morning as a substitute for coffee. Occasionally I take another in the afternoon for a quick boost. Is this drug as safe as coffee, as the label claims?*

A. Yes—if you're not overly sensitive to caffeine. A *Vivarin* tablet contains 200 milligrams of caffeine, about the same as two cups of brewed coffee. In some people, though, even a single cup of brewed coffee can cause side effects such as nervousness, irritability, and rapid heartbeat.

PROCESSED VS. NATURAL SODIUM

Q. *In your article on nondrug therapies for hypertension, you suggest that people with high blood pressure avoid salty foods. You listed some foods that are surprisingly high in sodium—including celery. Doesn't the sodium in a natural food have less effect on blood pressure than the sodium found in processed foods?*

A. Sodium has the same effect on blood pressure, whether it's consumed as table salt, in processed foods, or as it occurs naturally in foods. Some researchers have suggested that there might be a difference, but the weight of the evidence suggests otherwise. If you're monitoring your sodium intake, add up sodium from all sources. Celery does have more sodium than most vegetables (about 35 milligrams per stalk), but that's still not a lot.

RAW FISH: ANGLING FOR TROUBLE

Q. *How great a risk is there, if any, in eating sushi and sashimi?*

A. Raw fish may be contaminated with potentially harmful bacteria or with parasites, which can cause even more serious problems. There's a small risk that raw fish dishes may contain parasitic worms, which can cause abdominal pain, impaired absorption of nutrients, and anemia. Freezing the fish at minus 10° F for 72 hours destroys parasites, but home freezers may not sustain such a low temperature. For that reason, it's best not to prepare raw fish yourself. You can cut your risk by avoiding fish most likely to harbor parasites: carp, salmon, trout, cod, and Pacific rockfish.

Generally, it's safer to eat raw fish dishes at a restaurant. But there's no way to guarantee that the restaurant you choose —or its supplier—will have properly frozen and handled the fish destined for you.

TOO LITTLE IODINE?

Q. *Because I have a family history of hypertension, I do not cook with salt. Since most table salt is fortified with iodine, I am concerned that my family may not be getting enough iodine. Should we be concerned?*

A. There is no cause for concern. The recommended daily intake for iodine is small and easily met even on a low-salt diet. Shellfish and saltwater fish, as well as breads (which are made with iodized salt), provide significant amounts of the mineral. You'll also obtain trace amounts from almost everything you eat, since fruits, vegetables, and plants used for livestock feed are often grown in areas where the soil is rich in iodine.

TOO MUCH VITAMIN D

Q. *I'm postmenopausal, and a bone-density scan has revealed moderate osteoporosis. I've been advised to take 100,000 I.U. of vitamin D every week and a combination of Premarin and Provera. I also take 1,500 milligrams of calcium a day. What are the risks of this regimen? Is it effective against osteoporosis?*

A. Except for the vitamin D, your regimen seems appropriate. *Premarin,* an estrogen product, is effective in stopping further bone loss. Taken by itself, however, it increases your risk of uterine cancer. *Provera,* a synthetic progesterone-like medication, helps protect against that complication. Taking extra calcium is also beneficial if you don't obtain about 1,200 milligrams daily in your ordinary diet.

However, such a megadose of vitamin D is unnecessary and can cause calcium to be deposited in your soft tissues; it can also put you at risk for kidney stones and kidney failure. The usual daily dose ranges from 400 IU to 1,000 IU, depending on age and the estimated amount being supplied by diet and sunlight.

VEGETARIANS AND VITAMINS

Q. *I've recently decided to become a vegetarian. What vitamin supplements should I be taking?*

A. That depends on how strict a vegetarian you plan to be. If you eat eggs, dairy products, or tempeh (a fermented soybean product), there's no need for vitamin supplements. If those foods are not part of your new diet, you should plan on taking vitamin B_{12} tablets regularly. The recommended daily intake is 6 micrograms daily.

VITAMINS FOREVER

Q. *For several years, I've been taking supplements that include high doses of the B vitamins and vitamin C. Since you've indicated that vitamin supplements are necessary only in a few special cases, I may stop taking them. But I've read elsewhere that doing so can create what amounts to a vitamin deficiency. Is that true?*

A. No. Taking vitamin supplements doesn't create increased demand. And any excess of the B vitamins and vitamin C is excreted in the urine. When you stop taking supplements, your body will simply get its ration of vitamins the natural way—from the foods you eat.

WARNINGS ON DIET DRINKS

Q. *Some diet sodas and juices contain the notice "PHENYLKETONURICS: CONTAINS PHENYLALANINE." What is phenylalanine—and why the warning?*

A. Phenylalanine, which is an essential amino acid needed by the body, also happens to be a component of the sweetener aspartame. Most people needn't worry about the warning, but phenylalanine can be a problem for those few (1 in 15,000) who suffer from a metabolic disorder called phenylketonuria (PKU). Those people lack an enzyme needed to process the amino acid, which can reach toxic levels in their blood and tissues if dietary sources are not restricted. Accordingly, the FDA requires products with aspartame to bear a warning. Screening for PKU at birth is routine. Mental retardation can result if a newborn's PKU goes undiagnosed.

WHY NOT CANNED FRUIT?

Q. *Everything I read about proper diet calls for fresh fruit. What's wrong with canned fruit?*

A. Processing the fruit reduces the amount of certain vitamins somewhat, particularly vitamins A and C. And fruit that is canned without the skin has less fiber than fresh fruit. In addition, fruit is often canned in syrup, which adds calories. Still, canned fruit—especially when it's canned in its own juices—is a lot better than no fruit. Use it as a substitute for out-of-season fresh varieties.

HOW MUCH "CAF" IN DECAF?

Q. *I've heard that decaffeinated coffee has as much as 30 percent of the caffeine in regular coffee. Is that true?*

A. No. The decaffeinating process actually leaves behind only about 3 percent of the caffeine. A cup of decaf has 2 to 5 milligrams of caffeine, compared with 40 to 108 mg for regular instant and 110 to 150 mg for drip-filtered (an 8-oz. cup from Starbucks may contain up to 200 mg). You'd have to drink an enormous amount of decaf to feel any effect from the caffeine.

THE COLOR OF CARROTS

Q. *I eat a lot of vegetables, particularly carrots. Sometimes my skin gets a yellow tinge. I've been told that I should stop eating carrots when that starts to happen. Should I?*

A. Only if you don't like the color. While eating large quantities of foods that are high in beta-carotene—especially carrots—can color your skin yellow, that doesn't indicate any kind of harmful reaction. And it's totally reversible. In fact, you don't have to stop eating those foods altogether to make the yellow discoloration disappear; just cut back a bit on carrots and take up the slack with other vegetables. After a few weeks, your skin should begin to clear.

MOLDY BREAD

Q. *If there's a spot of mold on a slice of bread, is it safe to break off that spot and eat the bread?*

A. No. With a soft food like bread, simply removing the visible mold won't necessarily remove all of the spores. If ingested, those mold spores might cause gastrointestinal problems, such as diarrhea. However, you can safely excise a small moldy area from firm foods, such as hard cheese, salami, and some fruits and vegetables. Be sure to include at least a half-inch margin of safety all around.

FAT AND CHOLESTEROL IN FOODS

Q. *My nonfat yogurt lists 5 milligrams of cholesterol. How can a food have cholesterol but no fat?*

A. It's possible, but uncommon. Foods that have no fat—including most fruits, vegetables, and grains—generally don't contain cholesterol either. Nonfat yogurt and skim milk are among the few exceptions.

Many more foods, especially those that contain vegetable oils, have fat but no cholesterol. That's because cholesterol is found only in animal products such as meat, eggs, milk, and cheese. And that's why it's no trick for a bag of fatty potato chips or even a package of margarine to boast "no cholesterol."

FAT BEER?

Q. *Does beer contain any fat or cholesterol?*

A. No. The calories in beer (about 150 per 12-ounce can of regular beer and 100 for light beer) come from alcohol, carbohydrates, and a minuscule amount of protein.

HIGH-FAT INFANT FORMULA

Q. *I was astonished to see that coconut oil is a major ingredient in* Enfamil *and other top-selling infant formulas. Isn't that oil extremely harmful to the arteries? Why would anyone feed it to a baby?*

A. It's true that Americans have been advised to cut back on foods containing coconut oil and other highly saturated fats, which have long been linked to coronary heart disease. But at this time, those guidelines apply only to older children and adults. Babies under age two need fats to meet energy needs and to supply the raw material for cell membranes. Infant formulas contain 30 to 50 percent saturated fatty acids, about the same as breast milk.

IS BUTTERMILK FATTY?

Q. *How does buttermilk compare to plain milk in calories and fat content?*

A. Favorably. Commercial buttermilk is usually made by adding lactic acid to either low-fat or skim milk. (The acid sours and thickens the milk.) An 8-ounce glass of buttermilk made from low-fat milk contains about 2 grams of fat, which accounts for 18 percent of the 100 total calories; buttermilk made from skim milk usually contains less than one gram of fat, accounting for less than 9 percent of the 80 total calories, a negligible amount. By comparison, a glass of whole milk contains 8 grams of fat, or about half of its 150 calories.

MINIMUM FAT INTAKE?

Q. *We hear so much about the desirability of limiting fat intake to no more than 30 percent of calories consumed. But surely fat must play some vital role in the diet. Isn't there a minimum fat intake below which nutrition would suffer?*

A. Yes, but no one knows exactly what that minimum level is. Clearly, some fat in the diet is needed to build parts of the body's cells, particularly the cell membranes. In animals, diets with virtually no fat can retard growth and cause skin disorders. In certain cultures, however, people consume as little as 10 percent of total calories from fat with no apparent ill effects.

MONO- AND DIGLYCERIDES

Q. *Many food products claim to be fat-free but list mono- and diglycerides as ingredients. Aren't they fats?*

A. Yes. But they're added in tiny quantities, usually to keep baked goods soft. "Fat free" really means *virtually* fat-free—less than 0.5 gram (4.5 calories) of fat per serving, an inconsequential amount.

EAT MORE "HEALTHY" FATS?

Q. *I have a question regarding "healthy" fats. What are the best sources to ensure sufficient intake of essential fatty acids?*

A. Nutritionists have definitely identified two essential fatty acids—components of fat that cannot be manufactured by the body and thus must be obtained from food. These are linoleic and linolenic acid, found in seed and vegetable oils. Other possible essential fatty acids include arachidonic acid, which is found in meat, and eicosapentaenoic acid (EPA), found in fish and seafood.

Unless you've discovered a way to remove all the fat from your diet, you're probably getting more than enough of those nutrients already. Any attempt to increase your intake of fats, even "healthy" fats, is likely to do more harm than good.

Digestion and indigestion

EATING AROUND ULCERS

Q. *I have a duodenal ulcer. What foods and beverages should I avoid?*

A. The usual advice is to avoid foods containing substances that are capable of increasing stomach acid, such as caffeine and alcohol, as well as known stomach irritants, such as aspirin and anti-inflammatory drugs.

However, it is now known that well over 90 percent of duodenal ulcers are caused by a bacterium called *Helicobacter pylori*. A two-week course of antibiotics and an acid reducer can be curative in most instances and can also prevent recurrences, which used to be common.

BILE WITHOUT A GALLBLADDER

Q. *In a report on gallstones,* Consumer Reports on Health *explained that the gallbladder stores bile produced by the liver and sends it into the small intestine to help digest fats. But it didn't explain where the bile goes when a person's gallbladder is removed. Can bile still aid in digestion—and can it form stones elsewhere?*

A. Yes, and probably not, respectively. When the gallbladder is removed, bile will flow directly from the liver via the bile ducts into the small intestine, where it continues to aid digestion. Stones tend to form when chemically imbalanced bile is stagnant, as it is when stored in the gallbladder. They rarely form in the bile ducts, and never in the intestine.

FLATULENCE

Q. *I've recently begun suffering from flatulence. I'm 65 and have no obvious digestive problems. What could be causing this often embarrassing problem?*

A. It could be the food you eat. Rectal gas is the price some people pay for good nutrition.

Intestinal bacteria can ferment the remnants of certain

foods, thereby producing gas. Likely foods include bran and whole grains, as well as many fruits and vegetables, such as apples, avocados, beans, broccoli, cabbage, cauliflower, corn, cucumbers, melons, onions, peas, peppers, and radishes. Sometimes milk and other lactose-containing products (ice cream, puddings, custards) are at fault. Try cutting out suspect foods for a while, and see if it helps.

Swallowed air can also produce a small amount of gas. It may help to eat more slowly, chew with your mouth closed, and avoid gulping food. Over-the-counter remedies such as simethicone *(Gas-X)* and charcoal tablets are not very helpful.

Flatulence is usually nothing to worry about unless it's accompanied by a recent change in bowel habits such as constipation or diarrhea. That could indicate an underlying disorder such as an intestinal infection or tumor, irritable bowel syndrome (spastic colon), or poor food absorption.

HERNIATED ESOPHAGUS

Q. *My husband has had a burning sensation in his throat. It was diagnosed as a herniated esophagus, but I didn't understand the doctor's explanation. What is it, and what can be done about it?*

A. Your husband is suffering from reflux esophagitis, or heartburn—inflammation of the swallowing tube due to stomach acid coursing back up. Sometimes the problem is related to a hiatal hernia, in which the stomach protrudes through the diaphragm into the chest. It can also result when the sphincter muscle at the lower end of the esophagus doesn't close properly.

Your husband should avoid irritants, including alcohol,

aspirin, citrus juice, and coffee (caffeinated and decaffeinated). He should also avoid fats and peppermint, which tend to relax the sphincter muscle. He can help to reduce abdominal pressure by losing weight—or wearing loose-fitting clothes. And he should take advantage of gravity to keep stomach acid where it belongs by elevating the head of the bed on 4-inch blocks, and not lying down after meals.

Certain medications can help. These include antacids, such as *Maalox* and *Riopan;* acid-blocking drugs, such as cimetidine (*Tagamet HB*) and ranitidine (*Zantac 75*); and drugs that strengthen the lower esophageal muscle, such as metoclopramide (*Reglan*).

SORBITOL AND DIGESTIVE PROBLEMS

Q. *I've heard that sorbitol can cause digestive problems. Is that true?*

A. Yes. Sorbitol, a mild natural sweetener used in gum, candy, and many foods, is absorbed slowly by your digestive system. Because it remains in the gastrointestinal tract for up to eight hours, it may be broken down by bacteria in the large intestine. If you consume lots of sorbitol, excessive gas and diarrhea can result.

TEST FOR LIVER DISEASE

Q. *For several years, blood tests have shown that I have a slightly elevated level of the liver enzyme known as SGPT. But all of the other tests for liver disease have found nothing wrong with me. My doctor says it's not uncommon for a healthy person to have an elevated SGPT count. Is he right?*

A. Yes. Usually there's no known cause, assuming no lab error. (In obese people, it may be due to accumulation of fat in the liver.) If you've tested negative for hepatitis, including hepatitis C, you have nothing to worry about. However, your liver function should be retested periodically to make sure it remains healthy.

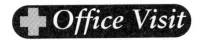

WHEN YOUR BELLY HURTS

Several years ago, I received two late-night calls within minutes of each other. Both callers were generally healthy men in their mid-forties. Both had diffuse belly pains, accompanied by nausea and vomiting. And both had had an appendectomy in the past. There the similarity ended: The first caller also had diarrhea and fever; the second didn't. Which one was sicker?

You might think the fellow with more symptoms was in worse shape. But that man's fever and diarrhea—two signs of probable infection—were actually good signs. By the next morning, his symptoms were starting to subside on their own. The problem appeared to be a case of mild gastroenteritis—an inflamed intestinal lining—which cleared up over the next few days.

The other man was in trouble. He needed emergency surgery for a blocked small intestine, caused by a band of scar tissue from his old appendix operation. Another few hours, and that segment of the bowel might have died, which would have meant removal of the dead portion.

Belly pain can be confusing. There are many organs in and around the abdomen. Any of those organs can hurt. And you can't always judge the severity of the problem by how bad the pain is, how sick you feel, or how many other symptoms you have.

Still, there is information that can help you figure out whether you should call your doctor right away or try to treat the problem yourself for a while.

PROBABLY NOT SERIOUS

The most common causes of abdominal pain are generally the least serious ones, even though they often produce disabling symptoms.

Gastroenteritis that stems from a virus, for example, can cause pain, nausea, fever, vomiting, and diarrhea. But the symptoms usually subside in two to three days. The most prevalent kind of food poisoning causes similar symptoms and runs an even shorter course, usually without fever. Both of those intestinal infections produce generalized belly pain, rather than pain confined to a single area. If the symptoms prove to be tolerable and begin to wane within a day or so, there's probably no need to seek medical attention. Just drink plenty of fluids and handle any pain with acetaminophen (*Actamin, Tylenol*).

Certain pain relievers, often used in high doses for arthritis, are another common cause of belly pain. If you develop pain in the central part of your upper abdomen while you're taking aspirin or an anti-inflammatory drug such as ibuprofen (*Advil, Motrin-IB*) or naproxen (*Aleve*), stop taking the drug immediately. The pain should disappear within a few days, with the help of an over-the-counter antacid, such as *Maalox* or *Tums,* or an acid-reducer like famotidine (*Pepcid AC*) or ranitidine (*Zantac 75*).

SIGNS OF DANGER

One clue that you may need immediate medical help is pain that's confined to one area of the belly. Such pain is more likely to involve a single organ than pain that's diffuse or that moves from area to area. And problems that involve a single organ are more likely to be serious.

Call your doctor immediately if you experience acute abdominal pain accompanied by:

• **Severe weakness, dizziness, or sweating.** All are signs of internal bleeding, either from the stomach or bowel or from a ruptured aortic aneurysm (a bulge in the body's largest blood vessel).

• **Bloody stools.** Possibly due to an ulcer, diverticulitis, a blocked blood vessel to the bowel, or telescoping of one segment of the bowel into another. Bleeding from the stomach usually results in black stools; rapid or lower-bowel bleeding turns the stools reddish. (Iron supplements and bismuth subsalicylate, the active ingredient in *Pepto-Bismol,* can also blacken the stools, while beets and cranberries can turn them red.)

• **Possible pregnancy.** Lower abdominal pain could indicate a spontaneous abortion or an ectopic pregnancy. (When not linked to pregnancy, acute abdominal pain in women of childbearing age can signal a twisted ovary.)

• **A bulge in the groin.** Likely caused by a strangulated hernia.

• **Chills and high fever.** That could signal peritonitis, a severe infection of the abdominal lining caused by rupture of the appendix, diverticulum, or gallbladder.

• **Pain spreading into either flank.** That's a sign of kidney stones, especially if accompanied by bloody urine.

With or without those symptoms, severe belly pain that starts abruptly and doesn't let up merits a doctor's attention. Even when belly pain is mild, you should still call your doctor if it persists for more than two or three days or recurs over a period of more than a week or two.

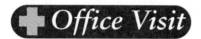

EASING IRRITABLE BOWEL SYNDROME

An aspiring young pop singer was telling me about a health problem that threatened her career, forcing her to miss rehearsals and even cancel a few performances.

Ever since she had returned from a gig aboard a Caribbean cruise ship six months before, she had been plagued by alternating bouts of diarrhea and constipation. She experienced abdominal pains before bowel movements, often felt bloated, and was embarrassed by gas. She thought she might have picked up some intestinal infection in the tropics.

But my patient also confided that she had had bowel problems before, especially at stressful times, such as during school exams or before an audition. A doctor once told her she had a "nervous stomach." She was afraid that I would label her a hypochondriac if I found nothing wrong with her physically.

I assured her that emotional factors could not be causing her symptoms, although stress or worrying about the problem could be making them worse. I'd check for parasites and other possible causes. But it sounded as if she had irritable bowel syndrome, a common disorder that afflicts as many as one in five adults in the United States.

DIAGNOSING THE SYNDROME

Doctors used to attribute irritable bowel syndrome to anxiety or depression. That was partly because people with the condition have no evidence of physical disease other than their intestinal symptoms and partly because anxious or depressed people are more likely to seek medical attention for those symptoms. Overall, however, there's no evidence that people with irritable bowel syndrome have more psychological problems than the average person. What actually causes the syndrome in the first place remains unknown.

Before I could diagnose irritable bowel syndrome in my patient, I first had to check for various underlying disorders involving the lower intestinal tract that can cause similar symptoms. Blood and stool tests ruled out any parasites or bacteria that she might have brought back from the tropics. A short trial on a restricted diet ruled out intolerance to lactose (the sugar in dairy products), which stems from a deficiency of *lactase* (the intestinal enzyme that breaks down the sugar). Careful questioning excluded a possible intestinal reaction to excessive amounts of sorbitol or fructose, often used as sweeteners in low-calorie products.

The other main possibilities were more serious: gynecological disorders, such as endometriosis; inflammatory bowel disease, such as ulcerative colitis or Crohn's disease; and even colon cancer. But her overall good health and normal blood tests suggested that she didn't have any of those disorders, so expensive testing was not warranted at that point.

I diagnosed her problem as irritable bowel syndrome and started treatment to relieve her symptoms.

SELF-HELP FOR SYMPTOMS

Irritable bowel syndrome can cause three different types of problems: constipation, diarrhea, and a combination of abdominal pain, gas, and bloating. Some people with the syndrome experience only one symptom; others go back and forth from one to another. Still others have the pain-gas-bloating complex plus either diarrhea or constipation at different times. Fortunately, most people diagnosed with irritable bowel syndrome can treat themselves, depending on their symptoms:

• Constipation is the most common symptom of irritable bowel syndrome. Note that a daily bowel movement is not necessary for good health. If you aren't bloated and you move your bowels without discomfort, you're not constipated, no matter how infrequently you defecate.

When constipation is a problem, extra fiber in the diet usually helps. That's because fiber absorbs water and swells in the bowel, creating bulkier stools that stimulate bowel contractions. People who are constipated should gradually add fiber to their diet over several weeks until they're consuming about 20 to 30 grams a day. (If you're eating more fiber, you should probably drink more fluids, too.)

Good sources of fiber include wheat bran, whole grains, whole-grain breads, and certain fruits and vegetables, notably raspberries, pears, peas, and brussels sprouts. Prunes are especially effective bowel cleansers, since they're not only high in fiber but also contain an irritant that rouses the bowel muscles.

If dietary measures alone aren't sufficient, a bulk laxative containing psyllium (*Metamucil, Mylanta Natural Fiber*) can sometimes help. But avoid regular use of other types of laxatives, such as saline products (*Phillips' Milk of Magnesia*) or stool softeners (*Colace, Surfak*). Over time, those laxatives can weaken bowel function. As a result, many people with chronic constipation become dependent on the drugs, which can have significant side effects ranging from potassium depletion to liver damage.

• Diarrhea, often containing mucus, is probably the easiest

symptom to treat. Again, dietary modifications can help bring relief. In this case, however, you should cut back on fresh fruits and vegetables that contain lots of fiber and eat more complex carbohydrates, such as potatoes, pasta, and white rice. If dietary measures fail, a few doses of over-the-counter loperamide (*Imodium A-D, Pepto Diarrhea Control*) will usually do the trick. Again, don't rely on medication any longer than you have to. (See your physician if you notice blood in the stool; that can signal a more serious disorder.)

• The pain-gas-bloating complex is the most distressing manifestation of irritable bowel syndrome and the most difficult to treat. A bowel movement usually relieves the pain, but cramps often return soon after. People who suffer from this set of symptoms apparently have increased sensitivity to normal amounts of intestinal gas. Even small amounts of food produce abdominal distention, or bloating.

The first step in treating this complex is to try to identify and cut out any foods that might be causing gas. The most common offenders include beans, brussels sprouts, cabbage, and onions. But the culprits vary from person to person, and you might have to do some detective work yourself. Some physicians recommend simethicone (*Gas-X*) or charcoal tablets, but I've found that those drugs usually don't help.

BEYOND SELF-HELP

If dietary measures and judicious use of nonprescription drugs don't bring relief, your physician can prescribe stronger drugs. For example, an antispasmodic medication may help people whose pain stems from intestinal spasms. But all you may really need from your doctor is reassurance that nothing is seriously wrong with you physiologically or psychologically. Irritable bowel syndrome almost always subsides on its own and often doesn't return for long stretches.

When I last saw my patient a few months ago, she had made several dietary changes and was coping with her problem successfully. She was less concerned about the symptoms that remained, and she had returned to the stage.

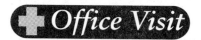

RELIEVING CONSTIPATION
—IF YOU REALLY HAVE IT

On a summer night in 1937, the boys in bunk six were getting ready for bed. Our horseplay stopped abruptly when the camp nurse entered, clipboard and pencil in hand. Muffled giggles punctuated the silence as she interrogated each of us in turn. "Hard, medium, soft, or none?" she asked. She wasn't taking egg orders —she was checking our bowel movements. Anyone foolish enough to answer "hard" or "none" was rewarded with a dose of castor oil.

Although that barbaric ritual has gone the way of public hangings, the obsession with daily bowel movements and the rampant overuse of laxatives continue. Bombarded by ads linking empty bowels to a full life, Americans spend about $300 million a year on the more than 700 brands of over-the-counter laxatives. Much of that money is spent needlessly, because of tenacious misconceptions about constipation.

One myth is that waste products can contaminate the rest of the body if they're not eliminated frequently. More than 60 percent of Americans believe that a daily bowel movement is necessary for good health. Actually, the frequency of bowel movements among healthy people varies greatly—from three a day to three a week. If you don't feel bloated and you move your bowels without discomfort, you're not constipated, no matter how infrequently you defecate.

CONSTIPATING HABITS

When constipation does occur, it's likely to strike older more than younger people and women more often than men. In some cases, it reflects an underlying medical problem: Constipation can be caused by hormonal disorders, such as an underactive thyroid gland; elevated blood levels of calcium; neurological injuries or disorders; or mechanical blockages of the bowel, such as hemorrhoids or tumors.

Usually, however, constipation is caused not by disease but by lifestyle and habits. The most common problem is too little fiber in the diet. Fiber absorbs water and swells in the bowel, creating bulkier stools, which stimulate the bowel contractions that push the stool along.

People who are constipated should consume about 20 to 30 grams of fiber a day. Eat them sparingly, or they can cause "rebound" constipation when you give them up.

Inactivity can also contribute to constipation. Jogging, aerobics, and brisk walking are good ways to stimulate the bowel.

Bowel movements are not just something your body does; you have to pitch in, too, by heeding the urge to defecate. Rather than rushing to catch the train right after breakfast—when the urge to defecate is often strongest—try to set aside enough time to let nature take its course.

A host of common medications can be constipating. They range from iron or calcium supplements and aluminum antacids to prescription drugs, including antidepressants, antihistamines, antispasmodics, narcotics, tranquilizers, and heart drugs such as calcium-channel blockers, diuretics, and antiarrhythmic agents. If you became constipated soon after you started taking medication, ask your doctor if drugs could be the cause.

CONSTIPATING LAXATIVES

Although the cavalier use of castor oil has declined, the myth of the benign, "safe and gentle" laxative lives on. Used regularly, all methods of purging the bowel—enemas as well as laxatives—tend to weaken bowel function and cause dependence. Research suggests that about half the people who use laxatives regularly could regain normal bowel function by discontinuing those drugs. And all laxatives can have significant side effects. Laxatives should be avoided if possible or used only occasionally.

Temporary constipation may crop up when travel or illness disrupts your normal habits, when there's a change in your diet, or when you're taking a short course of medication. The problem often resolves itself in a few days. If not, an enema or laxative can help. In any case, your accustomed bowel function will generally return when you resume your normal routine.

If you've been constipated for more than two or three weeks without apparent cause, consult your physician. After ruling out serious disorders, your doctor will help you design a program of dietary and other lifestyle changes. If that doesn't work, an enema or laxative may be required.

Doctors

D.O. VS. M.D.

Q. *What's the difference in training between an osteopath and a medical doctor?*

A. Doctors of osteopathy (D.O.'s) are similar to doctors of medicine (M.D.'s) in training, licensing, and scope of practice. The major difference between them is philosophical. Osteopathic physicians place greater emphasis on the role of the musculoskeletal system (bones, muscles, and tendons) in the healthy functioning of the human body. In addition to using conventional diagnostic and therapeutic procedures, they may use manipulation techniques to diagnose and treat medical problems.

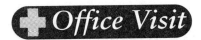 *Office Visit*

ARE TWO MEDICAL OPINIONS BETTER THAN ONE?

Not long ago, two patients called to ask if they should seek a second opinion before undergoing surgery. The first had a large aortic aneurysm—a severe bulge in the body's main blood vessel. A surgeon he consulted had recommended major surgery, despite the hazards of the operation and the prolonged recovery to follow.

The second patient had nasal polyps—benign growths that can contribute to congestion in people with allergies. An ear-nose-and-throat doctor had proposed removing the polyps with a simple surgical procedure that could be done under local anesthesia, with little risk and little pain after surgery.

WHICH PATIENT MOST NEEDED A SECOND OPINION?

Oddly enough, the second patient would have benefited more from another opinion. Caught early on, an aortic aneurysm can often be handled by lowering blood pressure and monitoring the condition. But for a large aneurysm, there's really no other choice but surgery. For nasal polyps, on the other hand, several nonsurgical options are worth considering.

I'LL SECOND THAT

A second opinion is even more important now than in the past. Under pressure to hold down costs, some doctors may suggest a less expensive course of therapy when another approach might be more appropriate. Or they may be motivated to boost profits with a more costly alternative. In some cases, doctors base their advice not on scientific evidence but on their own clinical experience or that of their close colleagues. Or their advice may even reflect their confidence in their ability to perform a procedure successfully. A second opinion is one of the best ways for a patient to be sure that none of those biase will bar the way to the best possible treatment.

Patients should *always* seek a second opinion on procedures about which experts often disagree. In addition to surgery for nasal polyps, some other common examples include cataract surgery or radial keratotomy; coronary bypass or angioplasty; ear tubes to relieve middle-ear pressure; hysterectomy; knee- or hip-replacement surgery; and surgery for a herniated vertebral disk.

Even when there are no therapeutic alternatives to sort out, a second opinion can be of value. It can offer a fresh perspective if there's a vexing clinical problem. Or it can confirm a diagnosis or the wisdom of a course of treatment, and thus ease any doubts you—or your physician—may have.

When seeking another opinion, try not to go behind your physician's back, since the second physician will usually want to review data obtained during the original workup, thus avoiding unnecessary duplication. If you sense reluctance or defensiveness on your doctor's part, that's all the more reason to get a second opinion.

HOW TO GET ONE

Your best guide to a qualified specialist is your primary-care physician. Ask for the names of at least two experts, preferably ones affiliated with a university medical center or a large, non-profit community hospital. Of course, if your primary-care physician gave the *initial* opinion, you'll need an unbiased source for a referral. That might come from a professional acquaintance—a doctor, nurse, or social worker—who knows a specialist personally or by reputation. Or you can call a reputable medical center or hospital and ask the secretary in the department that handles your type of condition for the names of staff specialists.

A referral outside your community lends independence to a second opinion by overcoming any financial or personal ties between doctors. Since physicians within a single community sometimes share an unjustified preference for a particular procedure, an outside expert may help offset local bias.

People in managed-care health plans typically find it harder to go outside the community. Such plans usually cover a second opinion only from an affiliated physician. Still, it can be well worthwhile even if it means paying for some or all of the consultation yourself.

Don't be surprised if the second opinion agrees with the first; that's usually the case. But if opinions differ, don't rush to a third source—you're not taking a poll. Instead, ask the doctors to support their opinions. Probe for answers to these questions:

• Have clinical studies shown that the suggested therapy will be effective? (Don't settle for anecdotal reports.)

• How will the therapy affect your quality of life if it succeeds? If it fails?

• What are the risks of the therapy?

• What are the alternatives?

• What will happen if you do nothing?

On rare occasions when the facts still aren't clear—or the first two doctors interpret the same facts differently—it's time to consult a third physician. Ask that doctor to explain why the first two disagree and to help you reach your decision.

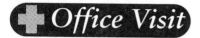 *Office Visit*

HOW TO SPEAK UP TO YOUR DOCTOR

A professor of mine back in medical school used to say that a carefully taken history alone could lead to a correct diagnosis about 80 percent of the time. But getting an accurate history is often easier said than done.

With some patients, the physician becomes more like a dentist—when getting all that information is like pulling teeth. And of course, many doctors—whether due to temperament or time constraints—don't pursue the patient's account as aggressively or even listen as attentively as they should. Either way, it's up to you to see that your story is told and your message gets through.

Do tell

Here's what to tell your doctor during an office visit—and how to tell it.

Tell why you're there. Especially if you have more than one reason for the visit, make a list in advance so you won't wind up kicking yourself on the way home for forgetting to ask an important question. Try to be specific when describing each problem. Saying something hurts, for example, is not enough. You need to describe when the pain began, exactly what it feels like, whether it comes and goes, and what makes it better or worse.

Tell what's bothering you most, first. Make sure your doctor realizes how important each complaint is to *you*. In one study, one in every four complaints mentioned by patients wasn't even recognized as a problem by their physician. In another study, doctor and patient disagreed about half the time on exactly what the main health problem was.

Tell it like it is. Don't minimize or trivialize your complaints, or your doctor may do the same. Don't attribute problems to "normal" aging—especially problems involving depression, dizziness, forgetfulness, or sexual dysfunction. Think of the nonagenarian who complained of knee pain only to have his doctor suggest that this was to be expected at the age of 92. "But my other knee is also 92," the man pointed out, "and it's fine." There may be an underlying, treatable disorder—at any age.

Tell it straight. Try to present your problems in a focused manner, without flitting from one symptom or complaint to another. Doctors tend to butt in quickly—on average, within 20 seconds after the patient starts talking, according to one study—so avoid rambling, which invites interruption. When your doctor interrupts anyway, remember to pick up the thread where you left off. Check your list to make sure you fully cover one problem before going on to the next. Also, since doctors tend to pride themselves on making quick diagnoses, make sure you get a chance to put all the clues on the table first.

Tell your primary-care physician all. I often encounter patients who are seeing several other doctors for problems involving various body parts. Such a splintered approach to health care runs counter to the concept of treating the whole patient and can produce disastrous results. Of course, there are legitimate reasons to go to different specialists for different conditions. But it's essential to keep your primary doctor informed about *all* the care you're receiving. That includes care from any "alternative" practitioners as well.

Tell about the drugs you take. Bring all of your medications—over-the-counter as well as prescription—to each office visit. Have your doctor check each drug against what's written in your chart. Discuss lowering dosages or even stopping medications you may no longer need or that might interact with other drugs. Make sure your doctor knows about any recent drug reactions you may have had, including allergies or side effects.

Tell about the "dietary supplements" you take. Just because herbs are "natural" doesn't mean they're safe. Like drugs, they can cause side effects or interact with each other, with medications, or with foods. Many vitamins and minerals, too, can pose risks, especially in high dosages. But although vitamins, minerals, herbs, and other dietary supplements can behave like drugs, they're not regulated the same way, and the risks—and the possible benefits—are still largely unknown. Even if you suspect that your doctor might not approve of your daily supplemental regimen, it's still important to provide that information.

Tell about your family. Your risk for many serious diseases—including cancer, coronary heart disease, and diabetes—can be strongly influenced by your family medical history. Be sure to keep your physician up-to-date on any recent illnesses or deaths.

Tell your end-of-life wishes. Keep your doctor, your lawyer, and close family members informed about the sort of life-prolonging care you'd want if you were incapacitated. But don't rely on conversations, and don't wait until you're faced with a terminal illness or, even worse, become unable to communicate: Make out a living will and appoint a health-care proxy now.

WHEN ALL IS TOLD

Of course, good communication with your doctor involves a two-way flow of information. So ask lots of questions—and be a good listener. Take notes, or bring a tape recorder or a second set of ears. Then, to make sure you heard correctly and to increase the chance that you'll remember what you heard, tell your doctor what your doctor just told you.

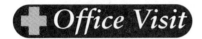

HOW TO TALK TO YOUR DOCTOR ABOUT SYMPTOMS

A few years ago, a 58-year-old social worker slated for elective surgery came to see me for a routine preoperative consultation. He had been having severe neck pain for some time. Two orthopedists had recommended surgery to correct a slipped disc.

I questioned him about his symptoms. He said that the pain, which radiated from his lower neck to his left shoulder and arm, came and went and wasn't linked to any sort of neck movement. Even more telling, his symptoms occurred only during the daytime, when he was most active. Since he didn't think that was relevant, he hadn't told the orthopedists. I sent him for a treadmill stress test. Sure enough, the test triggered the pain and showed that his symptoms were caused by coronary heart disease. He had his operation, all right—but it was angioplasty, not neck surgery.

HELP YOUR DOCTOR

Most of the time, a complete medical history can lead to an accurate diagnosis—even without a physical exam. But a lot rides on your ability to communicate your complaints to your doctor thoroughly and clearly. Here's how.

• **Make a list and check it twice.** Bringing a list of concerns to each office visit can be especially helpful when it comes to describing symptoms. So start preparing your list a few days in advance, if you can. Don't make the list too long; you don't want to put off your doctor with a three-page laundry list. But do be thorough. Omitting potentially important details or even jumbling the order in which your symptoms developed can lead to the wrong diagnosis—which, in turn, could lead to unnecessary testing or inappropriate treatment.

• **Speak up.** Since doctors tend to narrow their diagnostic choices very early into the office visit, you need to make your concerns known at the outset, before your doctor jumps to conclusions.

• **Get specific.** When describing symptoms, use the most descriptive terms you can. Think of analogies. For instance, don't just speak of "pain." Is it dull and aching, as from a toothache; burning, as from heartburn; stinging, as from an insect bite; piercing or sharp, as from a knife cut; or pressing, as if someone were sitting on your chest? Does it spread into nearby areas? How often does it occur? How long does it last? Is it affected by position, exercise, sexual activity, or emotional upset? What makes it better or worse?

• **Don't minimize your symptoms.** Remarks like "it's probably just gas" might lead your doctor to the same conclusion. Moreover, minimizing symptoms is often a cover-up for the fear that something is seriously wrong. If you worry that your "gas" might signal abdominal cancer, say so. A few reassuring words or an appropriate test could put your mind at ease.

• **Seek reassurance.** The week after comedian Gilda Radner died of ovarian cancer, I saw several women with lower abdominal complaints who wanted their ovaries checked. That's not unusual; symptoms often stem from fear of a disease that struck a friend or relative, or, in that case, a celebrity. But even if you suspect that's the cause of your symptoms, you should still talk it over with your doctor, if only for reassurance.

• **Tell all to someone.** Sometimes one minor symptom triggers a cascade of others that can obscure the initial problem. I recall one woman whose lightheadedness, sweating, and diarrhea led to myriad tests and ultimately to a psychiatrist. Careful questioning finally revealed that the entire alarming sequence was kicked off by a "skipped" heartbeat or two. Once that irregular beat was determined to be harmless, the woman's symptoms, caused by anxiety, promptly disappeared.

Occasionally, several symptoms form a syndrome—a constellation of symptoms that point to a single underlying problem—and the forest may be missed for the trees. I remember one woman who had her high blood pressure treated by a cardiologist, her backache by an orthopedist, diabetes by an internist, and thin skin by a dermatologist. It turned out that all her problems stemmed from an uncommon disorder called Cushing's syndrome, caused by a benign adrenal-gland tumor. That potentially fatal disease had gone undiagnosed—and untreated—for nearly five years because she had not discussed *all* of her symptoms thoroughly with one doctor.

HELP YOURSELF

For many people, the notion of modern medical diagnosis probably conjures up images of assorted high-tech tools, including sophisticated tests, computer analyses, and scanning equipment. To be sure, all those things can play an important role. But today as always, nothing is more important than the patient's own report of symptoms—and the doctor's analysis. When you make the most of your half of the equation, your doctor stands the best chance of solving your problem.

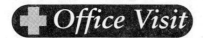

HOW TO TALK TO YOUR DOCTOR
ABOUT TESTING

Modern blood-testing technology makes it possibleto perform over two dozen tests on a single vial of blood in just a few hours. Since its debut in the 1960s, physicians and consumers alike have viewed extensive blood testing as an indispensable part of a routine checkup for healthy adults. Those tests were needed to catch disorders that might otherwise go undetected—and perhaps also to provide legal backup for the doctor in case of a malpractice lawsuit.

In recent years, however, managed-care organizations have been pushing physicians to perform less lab work. Medicare and many HMOs now restrict doctors from ordering lab tests unless disease symptoms have been identified or a diagnosis has already been made. The Preventive Services Task Force, an influential government panel of preventive-care experts, and the American College of Physicians also advise physicians to order lab work only when the results will lead to a life-saving finding or a dramatic reduction in sickness.

While largely a cost-saving move, the effort to curtail routine lab work does have some medical justification. More tests mean more chances of spurious findings, especially "false positives" that often lead to other, sometimes hazardous tests. And three years ago a Mayo Clinic study concluded that, for several types of routine tests, roughly 100 people would have to be screened to come up with a single test result that would lead to a change in treatment.

Though everyone agrees that lab work should be used judiciously, I believe that the current trend toward cutting back on routine testing has gone too far. Certain tests (including some not sanctioned by the Preventive Services Task Force) help diagnose diseases that can cause needless suffering or even premature death if allowed to go undetected and untreated.

REASONS TO ROLL UP YOUR SLEEVE

Listed below are the blood tests that I think should be part of a routine adult checkup. Unless otherwise specified, these tests should be done once every one to three years.

Fasting lipid panel. This blood test detects elevated LDL-cholesterol and low HDL-cholesterol levels, disorders that raise the risk of coronary heart disease and stroke. With proper treatment, however, those disorders can be controlled. Cholesterol tests help identify a significant number of people whose cholesterol levels require medical intervention.

Fasting blood-glucose test. This test identifies an elevated blood-sugar level, an indication of type 2 (adult onset) diabetes. The conventional wisdom used to be that patients with type 2 diabetes wouldn't benefit from early detection. But now we know otherwise, thanks to convincing studies showing that assiduously controlling the blood-sugar level can help prevent diabetes-related complications. And new diabetes drugs can control the blood-sugar level in nearly all patients with type 2 diabetes.

Liver-function tests. These tests can help detect hepatitis. Early detection may not help those with hepatitis A or B, since there is still no treatment for those diseases. But symptoms associated with hepatitis C can now be treated with the ribavirin-and-interferon drug combination (*Rebetron*). Whether that therapy saves lives is not yet known.

PSA test. An elevated blood level of prostate-specific antigen is a marker for prostate cancer. For years I've contended that all men should have an annual PSA test (along with a digital rectal exam) beginning at age 50—and at 45, if they're African-American and thus at higher risk. The Preventive

Services Task Force has argued that the test makes too many mistakes and that treatment for prostate cancer has not been shown to save lives. But PSA testing makes early detection and treatment possible, which may translate into a lower death rate, as is the case with mammography and breast cancer.

Thyroid-function tests (TSH and Free T4). Since thyroid disease may produce few if any initial symptoms, regular blood screening is necessary for early diagnosis. Early detection and treatment of thyroid disease can prevent heart arrhythmia, osteoporosis, dementia, eye disease, and premature death.

OTHER IMPORTANT LAB TESTS

In addition to blood work, three other types of lab tests should be performed as part of a routine checkup:

Urinalysis. This test checks a sample of your urine for microscopic amounts of blood, a possible sign of kidney or bladder cancer. Both diseases are best treated when caught early. A urinalysis should be done once every one to two years.

Cervical Pap smear. By examining cells gently scraped from the cervix, a laboratory technician can spot precancerous changes. If all women had regular Pap smears, almost all the nearly 5,000 deaths from cervical cancer in the U.S. each year could be prevented. Sexually active women should have a Pap smear every two years.

Fecal occult-blood test. In this test, a stool sample is tested for hidden blood, indicating possible colon cancer. An annual test, starting at age 50, can save lives by leading to the detection of colon cancer while it's still curable.

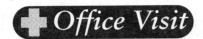 *Office Visit*

WHEN TO FIRE YOUR DOCTOR . . . AND HOW TO FIND ANOTHER

A 60-year-old attorney, a patient of mine for the past 15 years, sat across the desk from me and told me he was leaving my care. "It's not you," he said. "It's just that I can't be kept waiting. My time is just as valuable as yours."

I had good reason to be late that day, but further discussion was useless. This man had apparently been kept waiting one time too many. He had made up his mind.

And he was right. Patients shouldn't tolerate what they see as high-handed or inconsiderate behavior on the part of a physician—long waits, rushed consultations, perfunctory examinations, brusque or evasive answers to questions. Nor should they tolerate a condescending or authoritarian attitude, or a doctor who blames them when treatment fails. Patients needn't endure office staff who are rude or inattentive, or who consider it their job to shield the doctor from the patient.

Don't fire your physician in a moment of anger over an isolated incident, especially if the relationship has been a long and trusting one. Try discussing your grievances. Your doctor may not even know a problem exists. If the problem still can't be resolved, it's time to leave. Certain misdeeds, of course, shouldn't be forgiven even if they occur only once. Don't return to a doctor who misdiagnoses a significant problem or who fails to follow up an important abnormal laboratory result, for example.

FINDING A DOCTOR

There's no sure way to find a new personal physician who will meet all your needs. But a few steps can help you avoid a poorly qualified physician—and just might lead you to the right person.

First you'll need some names. Many people simply ask a satisfied friend or relative. A better approach, in my view, is to ask a health-care professional—a physician, nurse, therapist, technician, or social worker—who has seen many doctors in action. Almost anyone who works in a hospital can tell you which doctors are regarded highly by their patients and colleagues.

If you don't know an insider, call the local hospital and ask the medical staff secretary for the names of several family practitioners or internists on the roster who have agreed to take referrals for new patients. The county medical society can also provide names. Never rely on a paid advertisement in the newspaper or Yellow Pages.

Once you have a short list of candidates, investigate their qualifications. (If you have managed-care health insurance, see if your candidates are all "participating providers.") Look into these areas:

• **Education.** Residency training is more important than the medical school attended. Residency programs at big, typically urban university medical centers tend to provide a wider variety of cases and more hands-on experience than do those at smaller hospitals. If a physician holds a faculty position at a medical school, so much the better.

• **Board certification.** Medical specialty boards certify doctors who have completed an approved residency program and passed a test. A "board-eligible" doctor has finished his or her residency but has either failed or not yet taken the certifying exam. Your choice should be board-certified in internal medicine or family practice. An internist may also be certified in a subspecialty, such as cardiology or gastroenterology, which may be important if you have a particular health problem.

• **Hospital affiliation.** University and community hospitals, which themselves are evaluated by the Joint Commission on Accreditation of Healthcare Organizations, routinely check the qualifications and performance of their staff physicians. Your new doctor should be affiliated with a JCAHO-accredited hospital.

• **Professional affiliations.** Specialty societies, such as the American Academy of Family Physicians or, for internists, the American College of Physicians, exist mainly to offer continuing education to their members. Fellowship suggests the doctor has some interest in keeping up with the latest research.

HIRING A DOCTOR

How do you check for all those qualifications? There are several sources, none of them foolproof. It's probably best to consult one or more directories that you can find in a public library. Note, however, that none of those sources verifies all information provided by physicians, and some entries may be out of date.

Ultimately, you'll need to meet the finalists. Many physicians will see you for a brief introduction without charge. You're not looking for a best buddy, but you do want to avoid a personality clash. Once you've found someone you're happy with, schedule a checkup. That lets you check up on the doctor more closely, too. Does the doctor conduct a careful interview and a thorough physical exam? Explain all tests and procedures? Answer your questions fully and clearly?

Be sure to have your records sent to your new physician. Your former physician must honor your written request to forward your records. You needn't feel embarrassed about this. In fact, you might even let your former doctor know why you decided to leave.

Ear problems

RINGING EARS

Q. *For two years, I've had constant ringing in my ear that's gradually getting stronger. Tests by an ear specialist were inconclusive. What's going on, and what can I do about it?*

A. The cause of ringing or other noise in the ear, called tinnitus, often can't be determined. Tinnitus can result from almost any ear disorder, such as impacted earwax or infection. It can also be a symptom of anemia, cardiovascular disease, or Ménière's disease. Tinnitus is often associated with hearing loss.

Treating the underlying disorder, if one can be found, may stop the noise. If not, you can cover up the noise by playing background music or by using a tinnitus masker, which is worn like a hearing aid and makes a whining sound. Alcohol, caffeine, nicotine, and loud noises may aggravate tinnitus in some people.

EAR OF FLYING

Q. *Whenever I fly, I chew gum and yawn on both ascent and descent. Still, I experience pain in my ears, especially on descent. Afterward, my ears feel like they're "blocked" for the rest of the day. Is there anything I can do about this?*

A. Your problem probably stems from congestion blocking the Eustachian tube, which connects your nose and middle ear. When that happens, the change in cabin pressure during takeoff and landing can make the eardrum retract or expand, causing pain and impairing hearing. To keep the

Eustachian tube open, try taking a decongestant—preferably a short-acting nasal spray or drops, such as phenylephrine 0.5% (*Neo-Synephrine*)—shortly before takeoff. If it's a long flight, a second dose may be needed about a half hour before landing.

MÉNIÈRE'S DISEASE

Q. *What can you tell me about Ménière's disease? My doctor says there's no treatment. Is that true?*

A. The cause of Ménière's disease, a disorder that affects the inner ear, is unknown. Symptoms include vertigo (a spinning sensation) and tinnitus (ringing or other noise) in one ear or occasionally both ears. Gradual hearing loss often occurs. An ear, nose, and throat specialist can confirm the diagnosis with tests of balance and hearing. To rule out an acoustic neuroma—a benign tumor that can cause symptoms similar to those of Ménière's disease—a computerized tomography (CT) scan or magnetic resonance image (MRI) of the internal auditory canal within the skull should be done.

Treatment of Ménière's disease is usually not very effective. Strategies include diet therapy (usually low-sodium) and certain medications (antihistamines, sedatives, or diuretics). As a last resort, part of the inner ear may have to be surgically destroyed to provide relief.

LABYRINTHITIS

Q. *Several months ago, I experienced dizziness so severe that I couldn't walk or even open my eyes. I was rushed to a hospital, where the problem was diagnosed as labyrinthitis and treated with* Antivert. *Four months later, I still sometimes feel light-headed and have trouble keeping my balance when I look back over my shoulder. Will this go on forever?*

A. Probably not. Usually, each succeeding attack gets shorter and milder, although some people continue to have dizzy spells at irregular intervals for many years.

Labyrinthitis is an inflammation of the maze of inner-ear canals that control balance. The disorder usually arises from nasal congestion caused by a cold or allergy. The result is vertigo, a spinning sensation that disrupts balance.

Certain medications may help control the dizziness. These drugs include dimenhydrinate, sold over the counter as *Dramamine,* and meclizine, available by prescription as *Antivert* or over the counter as *Bonine* or *Dramamine II.*

✚ *Office Visit*

HEARING LOSS: DON'T SUFFER IN SILENCE

A patient of mine brought her 75-year-old father to see me. He'd become increasingly withdrawn and seemed depressed. He seldom spoke and often seemed to ignore people. His daughter thought he might have Alzheimer's disease. She questioned whether he should still be living on his own and wanted my opinion about hiring someone to care for him at home or placing him in a nursing home.

He did seem listless and a bit peculiar. He would answer some of my questions and then not respond at all to others. I soon realized that he was hard-of-hearing. He apparently tried to mask the problem by ignoring what he couldn't hear.

He said he'd realized his hearing was poor but had been ashamed to admit it, fearing that people might treat him like "an old man." Besides, he didn't want a hearing aid. He recalled friends saying that it made things worse by exaggerating noises and producing static.

After a long discussion, I convinced him to try a hearing aid. An otolaryngologist (ear, nose, and throat doctor) ruled out any reversible hearing disorder, and an audiologist (nonmedical hearing professional) fitted him with an aid. Several weeks later, his daughter told me he'd "rejoined the human race."

A SILENT EPIDEMIC

Such stories are all too familiar. Close to 30 million Americans —about one in three by age 65—have at least a mild hearing impairment. But people with hearing loss often fail to seek help. Some think that being unable to hear is just another unavoidable burden of aging, or that hearing aids might only compound the problem. Still others are deterred by the cost of the aids, which range from several hundred dollars to $1,500 or more. Only some health insurance plans pay for hearing aids; Medicare doesn't.

Because hearing loss develops gradually, a few people may not notice even a significant impairment. They may attribute their problem to people's mumbling, or dismiss family members' complaints about excessive radio or TV volume as just another form of nagging.

People who can't hear well tend to become isolated. Frustrated by their inability to follow conversations, they may stop trying and simply withdraw. Or they may make puzzling remarks that are unrelated to the conversation. It's easy to mistake such behavior for signs of depression or mental decline.

A DEAFENING DIN

Hearing loss commonly develops as people get older, in part because of the physical deterioration that accompanies aging. Very loud sounds, such as an explosion, immediately damage the delicate sensory cells of the inner ear. Chronic exposure to any sound that makes conversation difficult, such as the 85 decibels of a food processor, may eventually cause permanent hearing loss.

But noise isn't a threat only to older people. Loud music may be gradually deafening many younger people as well. A numbing 115 decibels—about eight times as loud as the food processor—can pour from the earpieces of a personal stereo. (On the decibel scale, loudness doubles approximately every 10 units.) And rock concerts can be even louder than the headphones—loud enough to do permanent damage in less than half an hour. Indeed, one study found that nearly a third of college freshmen already had detectable signs of hearing loss.

Here are some ways to minimize noise damage:

• Whenever possible, avoid situations in which you have to raise your voice to carry on a conversation.

• If someone else can hear the music coming from the headset of your personal stereo, it's too loud.

• Carry earplugs that you can use when you're exposed to blaring music, roaring motors, or other loud sounds. Inexpensive, compressible foam plugs that expand to fit the ear canal work fairly well. More expensive plastic plugs that an audiologist molds to fit your ear work better. If you're going to be around particularly loud noise, such as the whine of a chain saw, consider wearing an earmuff-style protector.

DETECTION AND TREATMENT

When hearing deteriorates because of aging or noise, the first sensory cells to go are those that pick up high-frequency sounds.

Voices may sound as loud as ever, but certain words become harder to pick up. Since some consonants have a higher frequency than vowels, certain words, such as "shin" and "thin," become difficult to distinguish. Background noise, such as the voices and rattling silverware in a restaurant, can make it particularly difficult to catch what someone is saying. Another early sign that may accompany hearing loss is ringing in the ears.

If you suspect hearing loss, don't just blame it on getting older. See your physician to rule out correctable causes. Earwax, for example, commonly builds up in the ear canal and can significantly reduce hearing. Over-the-counter kits for dissolving earwax may be worth trying, although there's a small chance that the loosened wax will settle deeper in the ear canal. Don't use cotton-tipped applicators, which can tear the ear canal or injure the eardrum. Any hardened wax should be removed by a doctor.

Hearing problems can also be caused by aspirin, nonsteroidal anti-inflammatory drugs such as ibuprofen (*Advil, Motrin-IB*), the heart drug quinidine (*Cardioquin, Quinaglute*), and other common medications. Reducing the dosage or switching to equivalent drugs can help. Some treatable conditions that affect hearing include circulatory disorders, inner-ear infection, hypothyroidism, otosclerosis (immobilization of the tiny bones that transmit sound vibrations), Paget's disease of the bones, and rheumatoid arthritis.

If there's no correctable cause and the problem affects your daily life—making you strain to catch what people are saying around you, over the phone, or at the movies, for example—a hearing aid can help. While today's devices still have drawbacks, they're a big improvement over the clunky, noisy contraptions that people used to wear.

Exercise

AEROBIC CRAMPING

Q. *About 15 minutes into my aerobics class, my calves begin to cramp. Why does that happen, and how can I prevent it?*

A. Aerobic exercises, especially those that involve bouncing, tend to overwork the large muscle in the calf. The cramping problem might be avoided if you varied your exercise routine to stress different muscle groups.

Always be sure to stretch your calves before and after exercising: Stand about two feet from a wall and place your hands against it. Bend one knee and move the other leg out behind you, keeping that heel on the floor. Lean forward until you feel the stretch in your calf. Hold that position for 30 seconds, then repeat with the opposite leg.

You can also help prevent cramps by drinking plenty of water both before and during strenuous workouts.

AEROBIC EXERCISE

Q. *Exactly what is it that makes an exercise "aerobic"?*

A. During aerobic exercises such as swimming, jogging, and cycling, the muscles demand a continuous supply of oxygen to burn the energy stored in their cells. That forces the body to improve its ability to use oxygen; this eventually benefits the lungs and heart by increasing the efficiency of breathing and pumping oxygenated blood.

Strength-training exercise, on the other hand, is usually

*non*aerobic; that is, the muscles derive energy from biochemical reactions that don't depend on oxygen. However, such exercise is equally important and has complementary benefits.

RESTING HEART RATE I

Q. *What is considered a "healthy" resting heart rate for a 47-year-old man, and how much can an exercise program lower that rate?*

A. A normal resting heart rate varies from person to person but is usually between 60 and 80 beats per minute, regardless of age or gender. With exercise and proper aerobic conditioning, however, the resting heart rate can be between 50 and 60 beats per minute. Highly trained athletes can have a resting heart rate as low as 40 beats per minute.

RESTING HEART RATE II

Q. *I've heard that your resting heart rate indicates how aerobically fit you are, and that a rate below average means you're in good shape. But when should you take your pulse to determine that rate? Mine normally ranges from the upper fifties after waking to the mid-sixties later in the day. When I'm tense and under pressure, my heart rate can soar into the upper eighties. Which of these is my resting heart rate?*

A. The best time to determine your resting heart rate is before you get out of bed in the morning (unless you had a nightmare, which could make your pulse race). The resting heart rate for a well-conditioned adult is between 50 and 60 beats per minute. So your waking rate in the upper fifties is admirable. However, a heart rate lower than 50 in anyone other than a highly trained athlete could be caused by a problem involving the internal rhythmicity of the heart and should be checked.

ROWING MACHINES

Q. *What are the benefits of exercising on a rowing machine?*

A. This is one of the best ways to exercise your entire body. The sliding seat works your leg muscles, and the rowing action works the muscles in your arms, shoulders, and back. It's excellent for aerobic fitness and for building muscular strength and endurance. Rowing is also a very good way to burn calories and increase flexibility. However, since rowing involves a fair degree of back flexion, those with recurrent back problems should first check with their physician.

SWIMMING FOR STRENGTH

Q. *I swim a mile six days a week. I don't kick as hard as I'd like when swimming because it makes my back ache, so I exercise my legs by walking 5 miles once a week. Is this an adequate workout for upper- and lower-body strength?*

A. The swimming gives your upper body a terrific workout. It tends to do less for your legs, especially if you don't work them hard. You might want to balance your upper- and lower-body workouts by swimming one day and walking the next.

WEIGHT LIFTING AND FAINTING

Q. *While working out with weights, I suddenly felt weak and started sweating from head to toe. I feared a "silent heart attack," but my doctor checked me on a treadmill and said I was okay. What happened? I'd like to avoid a repeat.*

A. You probably performed a so-called Valsalva maneuver when you were lifting weights: If you strain without exhaling, your blood pressure rises and your pulse drops. When you relax—as the weights are lowered—blood pressure can plunge and you're apt to feel faint.

Proper breathing while you're lifting weights is essential. Before lifting, take a deep breath and then slowly exhale as you lift. The same warning applies to the use of weight machines.

VARICOSE AND SPIDER VEINS

Q. *I've been doing high-impact aerobic exercise for the past 10 years. Now at 43, I've begun to notice both varicose and spider veins in my legs. Could the exercise be to blame?*

A. Probably not. Heredity, repeated pregnancies, and work that requires prolonged standing will all contribute to varicose veins. No one knows what causes spider veins—small, black or blue vessels in the skin of the inner thighs and lower legs. But there's no evidence that jolting exercise has anything to do with either spider or varicose veins. In fact, varicose veins are more common in people who are not physically active.

Eye care

CONTACT LENS INFECTIONS?

Q. *I recently read that keeping extended-wear contact lenses in place overnight leads to increased risk of infection. I have been keeping my lenses in for a week at a time. Is that unsafe?*

A. It may be. Extended-wear contact lens users are 10 to 15 times more likely than daily-wear users to develop corneal ulcers, which can become infected. In general, the risk increases with the length of time you wear your lenses, beginning with the first night's use. It is much safer to remove contact lenses daily, then clean and sterilize them each night.

HOMEMADE SALINE: SAFE WHEN HOT

Q. *Is there really any danger in mixing my own saline solution for contact-lens use? I make mine once a week.*

A. Homemade saline is safe to use only for heat-disinfecting your lenses. The heat kills any microbes that may contaminate the solution, which has no preservatives. Using homemade saline for other purposes, such as rinsing lenses, has been linked to a rare but severe corneal infection caused by an amoeba. The infection is difficult to treat and can cause blindness in the affected eye. In one study, 21 of 27 infected lens wearers had made their own saline.

DECLINING VISION

Q. *When a physician has determined that a 65-year-old patient has macular degeneration, does that mean eventual blindness? How fast does the condition progress, and is any treatment effective in slowing it down? Are there any support groups?*

A. Degeneration of the macula, a small, oval area near the center of the retina, impairs central visual acuity and color vision. The condition generally starts in a relatively benign "dry" form, but in more severe cases progresses to a sight-threatening "wet" form in which abnormal blood vessels under the retina leak, causing fluid to accumulate under the central retina. This process results in distorted images and blind spots accompanied by reduced visual acuity.

Progression of the disease is extremely variable, and the degree of visual loss depends on the location and extent of the damage. When deterioration is severe in both eyes, a person may become "legally blind": Reading is difficult, and driving isn't permitted. But peripheral vision is usually unaffected, and most daily activities can be maintained. In some cases, laser therapy can halt macular degeneration by sealing the leaking blood vessels. Some ophthalmologists recommend zinc supplements to stem the disease, but there is no hard evidence to support that approach.

The Association for Macular Diseases, which has a newsletter and a members' hotline, can inform you about support groups in your area. The address is 210 East 64th Street, New York, N.Y. 10021; 212 605-3719. The Lighthouse National Center for Vision and Aging can also refer you to support groups. Call 800 334-5497.

GLAUCOMA-DRUG SAFETY

Q. *Two years ago my doctor prescribed twice-a-day* Betoptic *eyedrops for incipient glaucoma. However, I've read that some glaucoma medications can affect the heart or lungs. Is* Betoptic *one of them?*

A. Betaxolol (*Betoptic*) is one of a group of medications called beta-blockers, which interfere with the action of adrenaline (epinephrine). That hormone, produced by the adrenal glands, helps control the heart rate and blood pressure. While beta-blockers taken orally can slow the heart and constrict bronchial tubes in the lungs, *Betoptic* eye drops are much less likely to produce those side effects. However, if you have a history of asthma or congestive heart failure, your physician should monitor you carefully to ensure that the eyedrops do not make your disorder worse.

OFF-THE-RACK GLASSES

Q. *Now that I'm over 40, is there any reason why I shouldn't use ready-to-wear reading glasses?*

A. Go right ahead, if they're comfortable. Store-bought reading glasses are perfectly safe—and they're quite inexpensive. Such glasses work fine for most people with presbyopia (farsightedness due to aging eyes).

However, you may need to switch to customized prescription lenses if you notice signs of eyestrain, such as headaches or tired eyes. Be sure to have an eye examination every two years or so after age 45 to ensure that your eyes stay healthy.

SPOTS BEFORE YOUR EYES

Q. *For several years, I've noticed small, gray spots in my vision. They don't prevent me from reading or seeing clearly, but they're annoying. My optometrist says there's no cure and not to worry. Should I do anything more about the problem?*

A. Your optometrist may be right, but you should still be evaluated by an ophthalmologist, a medical doctor who has more training in the diagnosis of eye diseases. The spots you describe are probably just harmless "floaters," but they could also signal other problems.

FLOATERS

Q. *Is there anything that I can do about "floaters," those harmless spots before the eyes?*

A. Try to ignore them. There's no treatment for floaters, which are actually stringy particles that form as the clear gel-like fluid inside the eye degenerates with age. Fortunately, floaters seldom interfere with vision and tend to disappear on their own. However, a sudden increase in their number or size, especially if accompanied by flashes of light, may signal a disorder of the retina, the light-sensitive tissue at the back of the eye. Eyes with such symptoms should be checked promptly by an ophthalmologist.

TWITCHING

Q. *For the past year, I've been troubled by frequent twitching in my left lower eyelid. Occasionally, the twitch extends down to the corner of my mouth. Eye exams have ruled out any disease, and my ophthalmologist says there's no treatment. Have you any suggestions?*

A. Such tics usually disappear spontaneously over time and generally require no treatment. Be patient. If yours are very annoying, you might seek a consultation with a neurologist.

PLASTIC SUNGLASSES

Q. *I've read that even clear plastic sunglass lenses block most ultraviolet light. Does that mean that my clear plastic prescription eyeglasses provide all the UV protection I need?*

A. Probably. Only people who are at high risk of developing eye damage need to wear lenses with a special coating that blocks additional ultraviolet light. This includes people who spend large amounts of time in the sun; those who have had cataracts removed without the insertion of an artificial lens; and those who take certain medications, such as allopurinol (*Lopurin, Zyloprim*), phenothiazine compounds (*Compazine, Thorazine*), psoralen drugs (*Oxsoralen-Ultra, Trisoralen*), tretinoin (*Renova*), or the antibiotics doxycycline or tetracycline.

Foot and leg pains

BONE SPURS

Q. *My foot doctor has advised surgery for painful bone spurs on the top of my feet. But I can't afford to stay off my feet for eight weeks. Would medication, laser treatment, or anything else relieve the pain?*

A. Bone spurs, an overgrowth of bone at or near joints (usually those of the big toe), don't cause pain; shoe pressure on the spurs does. Try wearing roomier shoes, stretch shoes, or extra-depth orthopedic shoes. Putting pads inside your regular shoes may help, so long as the pads don't put more pressure on the spurs. Aspirin or ibuprofen may relieve the pain temporarily, but that's not a long-term solution. Sometimes an injection of a long-acting corticosteroid (*Depo-Medrol, Hydrocortone*) can provide relief for months.

If those simple measures aren't sufficient, surgery to file down the protuberances may indeed be your best bet. Recovery from surgery rarely takes eight weeks, however. Most people can resume sedentary activities, such as desk work, within a few days and light walking without crutches or a cane in three or four weeks. So far, laser treatment for bone spurs seems to offer no advantage over traditional surgery.

FEET ON FIRE

Q. *I have a severe burning feeling on the soles of both feet. My circulation is normal, and soaking and applying powders haven't helped. Could this be a symptom of a serious ailment?*

A. A burning sensation on the soles of your feet can arise from any number of causes, from ill-fitting shoes to diabetes. The most serious cause is peripheral neuropathy—damage to the peripheral nerves—often from diabetes or alcoholism and less commonly from vitamin deficiencies or lead poisoning. A rare disorder called erythromelalgia increases blood flow to the hands and feet and can also produce a searing sensation.

Some people experience fiery feet because they're sensitive to a chemical in the inner lining of their shoes (particularly some types of athletic shoes). Try changing your footgear to see if the problem subsides. If not, see your physician to rule out medical causes.

MORTON'S NEUROMA

Q. *What can you tell me about Morton's neuroma?*

A. Morton's neuroma, a fairly common abnormality, is a benign tumor of a nerve in the web between two toes. The tumor causes pain when you walk or otherwise put pressure on the area. It may even feel as if a marble or pebble were inside the ball of the foot.

Treatment of the neuroma typically begins with injections of anesthetics or corticosteroids. Orthotics, special shoe inserts, can also help. If these measures don't work, surgical removal of the neuroma usually brings complete relief.

SPARE THE SCALPEL

Q. *I'm 72 years old and have a hammertoe and bunions on both feet. I'm in no pain whatever, but my podiatrist insists that I need surgery to correct the problems. What do you advise?*

A. You should change podiatrists. If the hammertoes and bunions don't bother you and don't hinder your mobility, then surgery is unnecessary.

SPINAL STENOSIS

Q. *For some time, I've had painful tingling in my legs, especially when I walk. My doctor says that's due to stenosis in my lower spine. What is that, and what can be done about it?*

A. As people get older, spinal stenosis—narrowing of the spinal canal—may begin to develop. Usually the canal becomes crowded due to the growth of bony spurs, a form of osteoarthritis. Less often, displaced joints and ligaments encroach on the spinal canal.

As the canal narrows, it can compress the spinal cord or the nerves that branch from it. That causes symptoms such as yours, as well as weakness and pain. For mild symptoms, nonsurgical treatments may provide adequate relief. Those treatments include aspirin, ibuprofen, or other nonsteroidal anti-inflammatory drugs; a spinal brace; and modified posture—leaning forward slightly whenever possible to decrease the pressure on the nerves.

Although those measures don't always work, they're worth trying before resorting to surgery. If necessary, a surgeon can remove parts of the vertebrae and anything else encroaching on the canal. Rehabilitation after the operation can take a while, but most patients eventually report good results.

TREATING SWOLLEN LEGS

Q. *I've had lymphedema in both legs for 12 years, and my ability to walk has steadily worsened. My doctor's only recommendation is an extremity pump to pressurize a sleeve that covers each leg. Are there any other treatments?*

A. Lymphedema is swelling of an arm or leg due to obstruction of the flow of lymph, a milky-looking body fluid. Leg swelling from lymphedema can be treated in several ways, but all treatments lose effectiveness over time. The "lymph pump" you describe can provide temporary relief early on, when fluid accumulation is less severe. The primary treatment for lymphedema remains the use of good elastic stockings. Various surgical procedures have been tried, generally with little lasting benefit.

WATERLOGGED LEGS

Q. *I am a 75-year-old woman. Last year my feet and legs became so swollen that I couldn't get into my shoes. My doctor said I had "water retention" and gave me a seven-day supply of Maxzide [triamterene and hydrochlorothiazide], which eventually relieved the swelling. What causes water retention, and how can I avoid it?*

A. There are several reasons for leg swelling. One of the most common is varicose veins, in which damage to valves in the large veins of the legs hinders the return of blood to the heart. Blood plasma, which is mostly water, pools in nearby tissue, causing swelling of the legs and feet. Excess dietary salt, sitting or standing for long periods, and hot weather can aggravate the swelling. Exercise such as walking or cycling helps. So does resting with your legs elevated. Water retention can also be caused by more serious problems, such as heart, liver, and kidney disorders. A medical checkup to rule those out would be wise.

Hair care

ESTROGEN AND HAIR LOSS

Q. *I'm a 67-year-old woman and have recently gone on estrogen replacement therapy for thinning bone. But now my hair is thinning. I've read that hormone treatment is a likely culprit. Is it?*

A. Actually, estrogen therapy is more likely to stop or even reverse the hair loss that occurs in many postmenopausal women. That's because the most common cause of hair loss in women is a combination of declining estrogen levels and simple aging. In addition, as female hormones dwindle after menopause, the small quantities of male hormones still produced by the ovaries cause further hair loss on the scalp.

If you're concerned about excessive hair loss, see your physician to rule out an underlying disorder that might be remedied. Possibilities include anemia, psoriasis, and disorders of the adrenal or thyroid glands. To safeguard what hair you've still got, treat it gently: Don't rub your scalp too vigorously; don't comb or brush too hard; avoid hot rollers and curling irons; set your blow dryer to low; and don't color, bleach, or perm your hair.

VITAMIN A AND HAIR LOSS

Q. *I'm a 42-year-old man with thinning hair. I've read that too much vitamin A can cause hair loss. Since I eat large amounts of vegetables that are high in vitamin A, could that be partly responsible for my problem?*

A. That's highly unlikely. While you could eventually suffer hair loss and other ill effects from taking supplemental megadoses of vitamin A, it's virtually impossible to overdose on the vitamin through the foods you eat. That's because the vitamin A in foods is mostly in the form of certain carotenoids—nontoxic vitamin-A precursors such as beta-carotene. Consuming large amounts of carotenoids can tint your skin orange. But that's not at all harmful, and it's reversible.

Thinning hair in a man your age is most likely due to male-pattern baldness, an inherited trait. Your physician can rule out other, uncommon causes of hair loss, such as an infection.

HAIR TODAY, GONE TOMORROW

Q. *Is there a safe way to remove unwanted hair permanently?*

A. Electrolysis is the only technique for permanent hair removal. A fine needle inserted into the hair follicle delivers an electrical impulse that kills the hair root.

Even the most skillful electrologist can have problems with

the technique. Applying too much electrical stimulation can scar the tissue around the hair follicle. Too little can fail to destroy the root. Rather than risk scarring, it's better to err on the side of understimulation and repeat the procedure, if necessary. However, doing so can become a prolonged, expensive process.

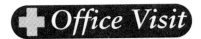 *Office Visit*

WHEN WOMEN LOSE THEIR HAIR

"It started about six months ago, and it's getting worse," a distraught 53-year-old stockbroker told me. "At this rate, I'm afraid I'll go bald in a year."

She had every reason to be upset. In a culture that worships a full head of "luxurious" hair, it's understandable that hair loss can be accompanied by a sense of emotional loss as well—especially for women. A balding man, at least, has plenty of company; a woman who's losing her hair may feel abnormal. According to a recent poll, about two-thirds of women who are experiencing hair loss say they feel less sexually attractive, compared with about one-third of men. And while a third of those men do nothing special to try to hide their hair loss, virtually all of the women do try.

Some hair loss is inevitable. But when a woman loses more hair than is typical for her age, there is often an underlying cause that can be corrected—or that will correct itself. If hair loss can't be reversed, you can still take steps to minimize the loss.

THE ROOT OF HAIR LOSS

To determine whether you're really losing hair faster than normal, count the hairs you lose during bathing and brushing every day for a week. (Use a strainer over the tub drain, and brush your hair over the sink.) The typical adult sheds about 100 hairs a day. If you consistently find many more than that, you probably are losing ground.

Every hair follicle goes through a cycle: It grows a hair for two to five years, rests for up to six months, sheds the old hair, and starts on a new one. Anything that shortens the growing phase or prolongs the resting phase will cause gradual hair loss until a new balance is achieved.

Many factors can upset that delicate balance. The most common factor involves hormones and heredity: In some people, the hair follicle in the scalp shuts down in response to male hormones. That response can cause both male- and female-pattern baldness. In men, the hairline typically recedes around the temples and over the crown. Women tend to lose hair more evenly, without developing actual bald spots.

In women, this hormonal sensitivity often shows up after menopause. As production of the female hormone estrogen declines, the small quantities of male hormones still produced by the ovaries are free to function unopposed. The same phenomenon can occur temporarily after childbirth or when a woman goes off oral contraceptives.

A wide range of disorders can also temporarily disrupt the growth-rest balance. Possibilities include a major illness, such as a heart attack; serious physical trauma, such as an auto accident; malnutrition; anemia; and disorders of the endocrine and thyroid glands. Certain drugs, especially chemotherapy for cancer, can also cause temporary hair loss.

Various other disorders can attack the hair follicle itself, sometimes leading to permanent hair loss. These include diseases that affect the scalp, such as psoriasis, discoid lupus, and fungal and bacterial infections, as well as an autoimmune disorder known as alopecia.

TREATING HAIR LOSS

My patient had already seen a dermatologist. He found no evidence of scalp disease and referred her to me. During my examination, I spotted no other possible underlying disorder.

I did learn that this patient had begun menopause about a year before. So her hair loss might have been caused by declining estrogen and a hereditary sensitivity to male hormones. If so, estrogen replacement therapy could have helped reverse the problem. But while such hormone therapy is warranted for women at risk of osteoporosis or coronary heart disease, thinning hair alone doesn't justify that treatment.

I told my patient that she could wait a few months to see if her hair stopped thinning, or she could try to regrow some of her lost hair by using the over-the-counter drug minoxidil. Sold under the brand name *Rogaine For Women,* it comes in a liquid or spray that you apply to your scalp twice a day. (There's now a more concentrated minoxidil product as well as the prescription pill finasteride, sold under the brand name *Propecia,* but those options are approved only for men and they're not significantly more effective.)

Using minoxidil means making a heavy bet on a long shot. In clinical studies, only about one in five women with mild-to-moderate female-pattern hair loss experienced at least modest regrowth. It can take many months for any new hair to be visible. If it works, you must use the drug indefinitely at an annual cost of $200 to $350. In some people, it causes itching and skin irritation.

And that's the approved treatment. None of the many over-the-counter remedies that have sprung up over the years has been shown to grow any hair at all. So they've been declared illegal, though enforcement is difficult. Bogus remedies to avoid include vitamins and other supplements, hair tonics, electric massagers and other devices, and anything else you might come across in the back pages of pulp magazines.

Surgical hair transplants are one rather drastic way to get hair to grow where it otherwise wouldn't—for example, where the follicles have been destroyed by scalp disease. The procedure involves moving small patches of scalp with healthy follicles to balding sites. That can be effective for male-pattern baldness. But it's harder to get good results in women, whose hair loss tends to be more diffuse.

Hair transplants can run as high as $15,000, and they're usually not covered by medical insurance. The whole process can take a year or two to complete, and it's painful. I recommend a high-quality hairpiece instead. While a good wig can cost up to $2,000, it's painless and the results are immediate.

HOLD ON TO YOUR HAIR

My patient decided not to gamble on minoxidil. Within a few months, the thinning stopped on its own. Meanwhile, I had given her some suggestions on how to treat her hair more gently.

Whether or not you're troubled by hair loss, here's how to safeguard what hair you've got:

• **Don't pull your hair.** When washing, don't massage your scalp vigorously. Dry your hair gently with a towel, or let it dry naturally. Avoid brushes or combs that pull your hair, and don't brush vigorously or any longer than you must.

• **Don't heat your hair.** Heat can weaken the hair shaft and even damage the follicle. Avoid hot rollers and curling irons. If you use a blow dryer, set it on low heat. Use a hat to protect your hair and scalp from the sun.

• **Don't use chemicals.** Anything that dries the hair weakens it. So don't color, bleach, or perm your hair. Wear a swimming cap to hold off pool chemicals.

• **Don't go on a crash diet.** That can result in malnutrition and throw off the growth-rest cycle.

Headaches

NOT TONIGHT—I'LL GET A HEADACHE

Q. *I sometimes get a headache during sexual activity. Your report on special imaging tests mentioned that as one reason to see a doctor. Why?*

A. To rule out the unlikely possibility of a brain tumor or aneurysm, which can cause headaches during certain types of exertion, such as coughing, bending over, straining during a bowel movement, or having sex. More likely, though, your headaches reflect muscle tension or vascular changes that occur as orgasm nears. "Benign sex headache," as it's called, most often strikes when the victim is tired, under stress, or having repeated intercourse. Some people first notice a dull ache at the back of the head.

If your headaches follow that pattern and a CT or MRI scan shows nothing wrong, you may be able to avoid trouble by taking a breather when you suspect an impending attack or by skipping sex during susceptible times. The prescription drug propranolol (*Inderal*) can usually prevent sex headaches, but it can also diminish potency or impair orgasm. Some people are helped by migraine medications.

ICE-CREAM HEADACHE

Q. *What causes the brief but excruciating headache you get when you eat ice cream too fast?*

A. Sudden, intense facial pain can follow the application of any ice-cold substance to the back of the mouth and the upper part of the throat. Apparently, cold triggers a reflex spasm of the blood vessels there. The pain may result from interrupted blood flow to the tissues. Similar pain can occur in sub-zero temperatures.

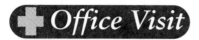

HEADACHES: WHAT TO DO AND WHEN TO WORRY

"When I see those flashing lights, I brace myself," a 33-year-old accountant told me, wincing at the memory. "Then comes the pain. I feel like my head is about to explode. I become nauseated. I vomit. I just want to die." She was describing the classic form of migraine.

Fortunately for her, there have been significant advances in migraine treatment in recent years. Other types of headache—including one that's even more severe than migraine—can also be treated. That's good news, since about three out of four adults suffer repeated headaches at some point in their lives. Here's my guide to identifying, relieving, and preventing the major types of headache.

Aching muscles

Most headaches are the tension type, caused by muscle spasms in the upper neck or just about anywhere in the head, including the forehead, scalp, or temple. The spasms are typically triggered by emotional stress or by holding the head in a fixed position, as when staring at a computer screen for hours on end. (In fact, I feel a headache coming on now.)

To relax the tensed muscles, try massage or a hot pack on

the neck and shoulders. Over-the-counter analgesics, such as acetaminophen, aspirin, or ibuprofen, often provide relief. If those measures fail, your doctor may prescribe muscle relaxants, such as methocarbamol *(Carbacot, Robaxin)*, or low doses of a tranquilizer, such as diazepam *(Valium)*.

Problems arise when tension headaches become chronic. Many patients get hooked on prescription medications such as butalbital, codeine, hydrocodone, or oxycodone, in combination with over-the-counter analgesics. Over time, those drugs become less effective and can actually cause rebound headaches as they wear off, leading many people to increase the dosage. Withdrawal can trigger severe headache—but that's often the only way to break the cycle. A better strategy for chronic tension headaches that don't respond to simpler measures is to try to prevent them with a tricyclic antidepressant such as amitriptyline *(Elavil, Endep)*.

THROBBING VESSELS

Vascular headaches occur when blood vessels in the head expand, causing intense throbbing or pulsating pain. The most common type is migraine.

Some migraine sufferers, like my patient the accountant, experience an "aura" before an impending attack. In addition to flashing lights, which can include blind spots, or numbness or tingling on one side of the face or body. In most cases, though, there's no advance warning. (Some people have only the aura without the headache.) Different things appear to trigger migraine in different people. Common possibilities include artificial flavorings and sweeteners, smoked meat, red wine, estrogen therapy, and the universal cause of just about all maladies—stress. Chocolate, too, has been blamed by many—though a study not long ago cast doubt on the connection.

Mild migraine may respond to nonprescription pain relievers. The FDA has approved *Excedrin Extra Strength* for treating migraines, enabling the manufacturer to package the old formula in a brand new bottle as *Excedrin Migraine*. The same product—a combination of aspirin, acetaminophen, and caffeine—can also be found in cheaper, generic versions.

For years, doctors treated more-severe migraine mainly with oral or injectable ergotamine *(Ergostat, D.H.E. 45)*, which has since become available as a nasal spray *(Migranal)*. Now there's also sumatriptan *(Imitrex)*, similarly available in all three forms. Unlike ergotamine, which generally works only if taken at the start of a migraine, sumatriptan can relieve pain after the onset, although its effects don't last as long. Two similar but longer-lasting drugs, zolmitriptan *(Zomig)* and naratriptan *(Amerge)*, are also available.

I prescribed sumatriptan nasal spray for my patient, who called it a miracle. To help prevent future attacks, I prescribed propranolol *(Inderal)*, a beta-blocker. Other preventive drugs include the calcium-channel blocker verapamil *(Calan, Verelan)* and tricyclic antidepressants. Limited evidence suggests that the herbal remedy feverfew may help, though its long-term safety is unknown.

Even more painful than migraine are "cluster" headaches, the other main vascular type. They usually last an hour or two, and can occur daily for weeks at a time before disappearing for long stretches. Inhaling pure oxygen can relieve the pain within minutes. Sumatriptan by nasal spray or injection can also provide relief. Various drugs—including ergotamine, verapamil, and corticosteroids such as prednisone—can help prevent attacks during the cluster period.

DANGER SIGNS

Occasionally, headaches can signal a serious underlying medical problem—such as a bulge in a blood-vessel wall (aneurysm), an inflamed artery (temporal arteritis), or a brain infection (encephalitis). A sudden, severe headache can indicate a hemorrhagic stroke. Headache can also mean a brain tumor—the worst fear of many headache sufferers—but other signs, such as seizures or a paralyzed limb, are usually apparent long before the headache strikes.

Seek immediate medical attention if you experience headaches that:

- Are sudden and severe or last longer than 24 hours.
- Get worse over the course of days or weeks.
- Get worse if you bend over, strain during bowel movements, or have sex.
- Are accompanied by weakness of a limb, loss of balance, or changes in vision or speech.
- Are accompanied by nausea and vomiting, fever, or disorientation.
- Are unlike headaches you've had before.

Health fears and risks

ALARM OVER SMOKE DETECTORS

Q. *The smoke detectors in my house have small print indicating they contain radioactive material. Is there any cause for concern?*

A. No. Ionization detectors use a tiny amount of americium 241, a radioactive element, to make the air in a small chamber conduct an electric current. Smoke particles entering the chamber disrupt the current, setting off the alarm. The risk from the minute amount of radiation emitted is negligible. Such exposure is roughly equivalent to moving from one apartment to another one on the floor above, and hence that much closer to the sun.

A far greater risk is relying on ionization smoke detectors alone to protect your family. Ionization devices respond quickly to open flames. But a slow, smoldering fire, the more common type of home fire, is better detected by photoelectric units, which rely on a beam of light and a light-sensitive photocell. Moreover, photoelectric detectors are almost as good as ionization detectors in responding to "fast" fires. When CONSUMER REPORTS last tested smoke detectors, the best performers were either ionization units or combination units with both a photoelectric and an ionization sensor.

FEAR OF FIBERGLASS

Q. *The fiberglass insulation in my basement ceiling is exposed. Because my wife's throat sometimes feels scratchy when she works in the basement, she won't let the children play there for fear the fiberglass is harmful. Is it?*

A. Probably not in this situation. Studies have shown a possible link between exposure to fiberglass and lung cancer, but only in workers who inhale huge amounts of the fibers for many years during manufacture or installation. Fiberglass insulation that is fixed in place usually doesn't give off airborne particles.

HEAT, HUMIDITY, AND HEALTH

Q. *I'm concerned about the unhealthy effects of heat and humidity in public places. What are the dangers?*

A. Heatstroke and respiratory infection. The risk of heatstroke becomes significant when the ambient, or external, temperature rises above 93° F. The risk of respiratory infection increases as the relative humidity falls below 20 percent. For health and comfort, ambient temperatures of 65° to 75° F and humidity levels of 30 to 40 percent are ideal.

NORMAL BODY TEMPERATURE

Q. *My temperature never seems to reach the "normal" level of 98.6° F. In fact, I rarely get a reading much higher than 97.5° or so, unless I'm sick. Is this unusual?*

A. Not at all. The time-honored "normal" oral temperature of 98.6° F represented the average for healthy people, and that number has been revised downward to 98.2°. Some perfectly healthy people never break 98.0°. In addition, your normal body temperature can vary, depending in part on the time of day: It's consistently lowest in the morning and highest in the late afternoon or evening. That daily variation can range anywhere from about 0.7° to 2.6° F.

✚ *Office Visit*

SUBTLE SYMPTOMS
THAT SIGNAL DANGER

After nearly a year of increasing constipation and two miserable days of repeated vomiting, a 75-year-old retired firefighter came to see me at the insistence of his wife. On examination,

I found evidence of acute intestinal obstruction and chronic weight loss. Suspecting colon cancer, I immediately admitted him to the hospital for further work-up.

There, my suspicions were confirmed: The tumor had completely encircled a segment of his intestine, narrowing it to the point that virtually no fecal matter was able to pass. Emergency surgery relieved the obstruction. But by then it was too late. The cancer had already spread to his liver. He died six months later.

OMINOUS, NOT ALWAYS OBVIOUS

If only he'd known how to read the early warning signs, there would have been a better chance of curing his cancer. But he mistakenly blamed his progressively narrowing stools on his enlarged prostate gland. He attributed his increasing constipation to having eaten less of late. And he figured that's why he was losing weight.

Unpleasant symptoms of one sort or another are the body's way of letting you know that something is wrong. Most people don't think twice about calling the doctor when they're in pain or running a high fever. But there's less motivation to seek medical help when you're not uncomfortable or worried. And indeed, most minor annoyances can be safely ignored, especially if they subside on their own. But some commonplace symptoms that are commonly ignored can signal real danger. Here are a few warning signs to watch out for:

• **Bowel changes.** Most people would dismiss an occasional bout of stomach upset—such as bloating, cramps, and constipation—as the result of something they ate. And various foods or temporary changes in eating habits can indeed cause such symptoms. However, as in the case of my unfortunate patient, altered bowel habits that persist and worsen can also signal colorectal cancer. Ovarian cancer can be heralded by similar symptoms. Basically, any change of bowel habits that doesn't disappear over a period of several weeks warrants a visit to the doctor.

• **Rectal bleeding.** People with hemorrhoids may sometimes pass blood in their stool. So it's easy to dismiss rectal bleeding as just another hemorrhoidal flare-up. But it can also signal benign or malignant polyps. Whatever the cause—even if it turns out to be nothing more than hemorrhoids—rectal bleeding on more than one occasion within a few weeks deserves medical attention.

• **Weight loss.** Most overweight people would probably be delighted to lose weight without trying. But weight loss that can't be explained by diet and exercise may be an early sign of conditions such as diabetes, an overactive thyroid gland, or poor absorption of nutrients from the intestinal tract. Those disorders can all cause you to lose weight even if you're eating more than usual. If you happen to be dieting, the extra weight loss may be mistaken for a sign of success.

• **Itching.** What may seem like an innocent itch can actually be an ominous symptom, especially if there's no rash or any other sign of skin irritation. It's easy to dismiss such itching as "winter skin," brought on by dry air, but if the itching is worse than you've experienced in previous years—or if it's not winter—an underlying disorder may be to blame. Possibilities range from diabetes, iron-deficiency anemia, and an overactive thyroid to more dire diseases, including leukemia, lymphomas, and cancer of the gallbladder, intestinal tract, or liver.

• **Leg pains.** Tired, achy legs can be brought on by a long day at the mall. But if even a short walk when you're well rested causes leg pain, it could be something more serious. If the pain is limited to one calf, it could be a sign of narrowing of the blood vessels due to arteriosclerosis. If you have pain in both legs, it could be due to spinal stenosis, an overgrowth of bony tissue that compresses the nerves in the lower spine .

• **Red stretch marks.** Ordinary stretch marks, which usually appear on the abdomen, flanks, and breasts, are permanent signs of rapid weight gain, often due to pregnancy. Those pale or silvery areas of thinned skin are at worst a cosmetic concern. But stretch marks that are red or purplish may indicate Cushing's disease, a disorder in which the adrenal glands produce too much of the hormone cortisol, thinning the skin and bones and increasing the risk of infection. Such stretch marks are especially likely to signal Cushing's disease in people who also have the triad of diabetes, hypertension, and osteoporosis.

WHEN TO CALL THE DOCTOR

That rundown of seemingly benign symptoms shouldn't frighten you into calling your doctor every time you sneeze. There are a few basic guidelines that can help you decide whether to seek medical attention.

A symptom you might be tempted to ignore should be taken seriously if it:

• Represents a sudden change from your usual patterns of symptoms.

• Persists for more than two or three weeks.

• Gradually gets worse.

• Interferes with your daily routine.

• Seems like an exaggerated version of a familiar symptom that you had previously been able to explain.

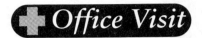 *Office Visit*

SYMPTOMS THAT ARE SCARY BUT NOT SERIOUS

A few months ago, a worried middle-aged accountant made an emergency visit to my office. He had passed a black stool earlier that day and was sure he was bleeding internally. He feared he had colon cancer. A digital rectal exam revealed a black stool all right, but the test for blood was negative. The culprit turned out to be bismuth subsalicylate—*Pepto-Bismol*—which he had taken the previous night for an upset stomach. His stool color was back to normal the next day.

Pepto-Bismol is not the only cause of needless worry about abnormally colored stools. A generous serving of beets, for example, which imparts a dark red color to feces, can also be troubling to the unsuspecting. Iron supplements, too, can blacken the stool.

ASSUME THE BEST

Passing a discolored stool is just one example of an apparent symptom that can be alarming yet medically insignificant. Here are a few common conditions that send patients running to the doctor when all that's needed is minimal attention or simple reassurance.

• **Red-eye special.** Subconjunctival hemorrhage sounds horrendous and looks even worse. One eye suddenly becomes blood-red due to a leaky blood vessel in the conjunctiva, the delicate transparent membrane that covers the white of the eye. That can be caused by just about any effort that temporarily increases pressure in the head—coughing, sneezing, bending over, lifting weights, straining during a bowel movement, or even orgasm.

Despite its appearance, subconjunctival hemorrhage is painless and harmless, and it doesn't even interfere with vision. The blood is slowly reabsorbed and disappears over the next few weeks.

• **Yellowed skin.** You might be upset if you noticed that your skin had turned orangy yellow. Could it be jaundice, the result of excess bile in the blood due to hepatitis or some other disease? If the whites of your eyes aren't turning yellow, too, the skin discoloration, called carotenemia, just means you've been eating lots of carrots or else taking supplements containing beta-carotene.

Carotenemia is the medical term for increased blood levels of the pigment carotene, a vitamin-A precursor found mainly in fruits and vegetables, especially carrots and sweet potatoes. The excess carotene is deposited in the skin, where it imparts that distinctive hue. High blood levels of carotene are harmless; enzymes in the body limit that nutrient's conversion to vitamin A so the vitamin won't reach toxic levels. If you don't like the color, cut down on the carrots or supplements. Your skin color will return to normal after a few weeks.

• **"Sighing" respirations,** a type of abnormal breathing, often causes great anxiety. Ironically, the condition is caused by underlying anxiety in the first place. Although it can be worrisome to the sufferer, the problem has nothing to do with the lungs.

Typically, the patient complains of a frustrated effort to inhale deeply. It's as if you had been interrupted halfway through a yawn. The distressing sensation may occur several times an hour. But tests of pulmonary function and breathing rhythm will detect nothing abnormal.

Since sighing respirations thrive on anxiety, they often subside once the patient has been reassured that there's no medical problem. If they don't go away, the underlying anxiety should be treated.

• **Low blood pressure.** Patients sometimes seek advice because they're worried that their blood pressure is too low. They may have tried out a relative's home monitor or had their pressure tested at the local supermarket. In fact, many perfectly healthy people—especially short, slim women—have systolic readings (the "upper" number) of less than 100 mm Hg, well below the usual "optimal" level of 120 mm Hg. So long as you're feeling fine and don't get lightheaded when you get up from lying or sitting down, your "low blood pressure" is no cause for concern. On the contrary, it's good for the cardiovascular system, since it puts less stress on the blood vessels.

• **Painful breastbone.** I often see patients who are troubled by this mysterious symptom, especially during the summer months or after they return from a tropical vacation in the winter. Out of nowhere, it seems, a painful lump develops at the lower end of the breastbone. Actually, the "lump" is just the normal cartilage that's suddenly noticeable only because it's sore. The victim has invariably been lying belly down for long relaxing hours on the sand. The sensitivity subsides within a few days if you avoid that prone position.

IGNORANCE IS NOT BLISS

With his discolored stool traced to the *Pepto-Bismol*, my patient felt immensely relieved, if a bit sheepish—especially since the product label clearly warns about that probable side effect.

Still, it's a good idea at least to call your doctor the first time unusual signs or symptoms develop. But don't assume the worst. Often, reassurance is the only treatment that's needed. And your new understanding could spare you needless worry in the future.

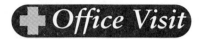

GENETIC TESTING: DO YOU REALLY WANT TO KNOW?

When I was a third-year medical student, I couldn't wait to listen to hearts, palpate bellies, and tap reflexes. But my classmates and I were restrained from using our stethoscopes and reflex hammers until we became adept at the art of talking to the patient. We soon learned that a complete medical history could predict a diagnosis in eight out of ten cases, and that an integral part of that medical history was the family history.

In the years since, advances in genetics have made detailed family history more important than ever. But not all doctors nowadays have the time or the interest to review their patients' family history. In one study evaluating the medical records of patients at a university-based clinic, only 13 percent of the records noted a positive family history for alcohol problems, whereas telephone interviews with the patients found that 40 percent reported a family history of alcoholism. If your physician doesn't ask about diseases that run in your family, be sure to speak up.

SHOULD YOU SCREEN YOUR GENES?

Not long ago, a 39-year-old woman informed me that her sister recently underwent a mastectomy for breast cancer. Knowing that the disease runs in families, this woman wondered whether she and her mother should be tested for a BRCA1 and BRCA2 gene mutation. If that defect is found, their chances of eventually developing breast cancer would rise to as much as 85 percent, and their risk of ovarian cancer would climb to nearly 30 percent. What would I advise?

My advice for everyone considering genetic testing is first

to undergo genetic counseling. Genetic counselors are trained to analyze your family history and evaluate your risk of developing or passing along an inherited disease. They can also help you determine whether testing is warranted. Genetic tests are only for people whose family history puts them at especially high risk of having a genetic defect. And even high-risk individuals don't always obtain conclusive answers or greater peace of mind.

In my patient's case, for example, both she and her mother tested positive for the mutated gene. My patient took the news well, and she's resolved to make regular breast-cancer screenings a priority. Her mother reacted very differently: She blamed herself for passing the gene to her daughters, and she may now need psychological therapy to cope with her guilt feelings.

SEEKING WISE COUNSEL

If you opt for genetic counseling, the counselor you work with should have at least a master's degree in genetic counseling, plus certification by the American Board of Medical Genetics or the American Board of Genetic Counseling. The National Society of Genetic Counselors can give you the names of genetic counselors in your area. You can also find a counselor by contacting a local hospital or the nearest university-affiliated hospital or medical school. Be prepared to do your own legwork rather than count on your doctor for a referral. According to a recent survey, 20 percent of internists in one state weren't even aware whether genetic counseling was available in their area.

Genetic counseling is advisable if:

• Your family history indicates a suspicious pattern of disease involving immediate blood relatives (parents, siblings, and children) or other close kin (grandparents, aunts, uncles, and first cousins).

• You're planning to become pregnant and are at increased risk of passing a genetic disorder to your baby. Individuals at increased risk include women who conceive at age 34 or older; individuals with a known genetic disorder; parents who've previously given birth to a child with a genetic defect; and members of certain ethnic groups with an increased incidence of an inherited disease.

If genetic testing seems to make sense in your case, be sure to think through the drawbacks as well as the benefits before making a decision.

THE BENEFITS OF TESTING

• **You can stop worrying.** Learning that you don't carry the family curse can take a load off your mind. A negative result can also save your relatives needless screening tests.

• **You can stay vigilant.** A positive result can motivate you to seek more frequent screenings for signs of the disease at an early, treatable stage. It may also prompt you to try reducing risk factors within your control, such as smoking or obesity.

• **You'll be better prepared.** If the news is not good, and a bad disease is inevitable, you'll have the opportunity to do some advance planning, such as having your children checked, taking those trips you always wanted to take, or perhaps writing your memoirs.

THE DRAWBACKS OF TESTING

• **You may not be able to do anything about the results.** Simply knowing that your family history puts you at high risk for a disease should provide ample incentive for intensified prevention or screening. However, for some diseases there may be little or nothing you can do.

• **You'd still worry.** Having a genetic defect doesn't mean you'll necessarily get the disease; depending on the defect and

the disease, your risk may range anywhere from slightly higher than normal to virtual certainty. Either way, the test result
can be emotionally devastating. It can push some people into
depression, which can then pose a greater threat than the
genetic disorder itself.

• **You risk discrimination.** Medical secrets are hard to keep;
employers or insurers have ways of finding out. Some states
have passed antidiscrimination laws, but such protection is
not foolproof.

Hernias

LASERS FOR HERNIA REPAIR

Q. *I expect to need surgery for a hernia. Is the new laser
technique better than a conventional operation?*

A. Not necessarily. When part of the intestine "herniates"
through the muscles of the abdominal wall, a surgeon must
reposition the herniated segment and reinforce the weakened
muscle. But the incision is the same whether the surgeon uses
a scalpel or a laser. Both procedures are performed under local
anesthesia on an outpatient basis. Some surgeons use lasers to
"weld" the wall of the abdomen shut; but that weak bond still
has to be reinforced by sutures, and the method won't make
you heal any faster.

UMBILICAL RUPTURE

Q. *My 48-year-old husband's doctor recommends surgical repair for an umbilical rupture. But it's not causing any discomfort now, and other doctors never noticed it. Is surgery really necessary?*

A. Perhaps not. An umbilical (belly button) rupture, or hernia, is caused by weakness or separation of the abdominal muscle fibers near the navel. When you stand, cough, or strain, the hernia becomes apparent: A portion of the intestine pushes through the muscle and appears as a bulge under the skin. Most of the time, the intestine can be put back into place if the person lies down and gently presses against the bulge. Such hernias are usually congenital but may not be detected until middle age.

Surgery can prevent "strangulation"—impaired blood flow to a trapped portion of intestine—but strangulation isn't likely anyway. If your husband remains free of pain and the bulge doesn't bother him, he may be able to do without an operation. However, if pain develops, he should return to his physician and reconsider surgery.

Immunizations

ADULT IMMUNIZATIONS

Q. *How often do adults need to have a tetanus shot or any other routine shots?*

A. All adults should receive a tetanus-diphtheria toxoid booster every 10 years. If an injury that might lead to tetanus occurs more than five years after the last shot, another booster should be given. (The next shot would then be given 10 years from that date.) People age 65 or over and those in certain high-risk groups should receive pneumococcal vaccine once and influenza vaccine annually.

JUST ONE SHOT FOR PNEUMONIA?

Q. *You've said that people 65 and older should receive pneumococcal vaccine just once. But some doctors have told me they recommend the shot every five years. I had one six years ago when I was 71. Should I get another?*

A. Healthy older people generally need only one dose of pneumococcal vaccine. (However, a single revaccination with the "23-valent" vaccine is worth considering if you previously received the older "14-valent" type of pneumococcal vaccine.) However, if you have a medical condition such as heart, kidney, liver, or lung disease, diabetes, Hodgkin's disease, cerebrospinal fluid leaks, an immune system disorder, or sickle-cell anemia, you could be susceptible to complications from pneumonia. Anyone in those risk groups should get a shot every six years.

FLU SHOTS

Q. *I've heard so many opinions, pro and con, about flu shots. Who should get a flu shot? How effective is it? When is the best time to get one?*

A. Anyone who can tolerate a flu shot should consider getting one before the influenza season begins. That's especially important for these high-risk groups:

• People age 65 or over.

• People with chronic lung or heart disorders, including children with asthma.

• Adults and children who during the preceding year needed regular medical care or hospitalization for a chronic disease: diabetes, kidney disorders, sickle-cell disease, or suppressed immune systems (including HIV/AIDS).

• Children and teenagers 6 months to 18 years who are on long-term aspirin therapy.

• People who live with or care for a person at high risk. A flu shot takes about two weeks to provide protection and lasts about six months. But the injection does not provide full immunity in all cases. It's about 90 percent effective in young, healthy people, and 70 percent effective in elderly, high-risk people—for the strains of influenza included in the vaccine. If an unexpected strain of flu pops up during the flu season, the vaccine may not work at all.

Generally, October is the best time for a flu shot, but any time between September and February is better than not at all. Travelers abroad, however, should consider a flu shot whatever the month. They may risk exposure to the virus at any time of year.

CAN YOU TOLERATE A FLU SHOT?

Q. *You say that "anyone who can tolerate a flu shot" should consider getting one. Exactly who can't tolerate a flu shot?*

A. People allergic to eggs, which are used to make the influenza vaccine, should not receive the shot. And people with an acute illness, such as a respiratory, gastrointestinal, or urinary-tract infection, should wait until they recover. Pregnant women should delay a flu shot until after the first trimester, unless they are at high risk.

Men's health

PROSTATE PROBLEMS

Q. *Can urinary or sexual habits affect the incidence or severity of an enlarged prostate or any other prostate problems?*

A. Those personal habits have nothing to do with the development of any prostate problems. However, modifying certain habits may help reduce the severity of symptoms. For example, urinating more frequently to keep the bladder from overfilling, allowing enough time to empty the bladder completely, and cutting back on fluids for several hours before bedtime can help reduce symptoms from an enlarged prostate. And since congestion in the prostate gland can aggravate the discomfort from chronic prostatitis (inflammation often due to bacterial infection), many urologists recommend frequent ejaculations to minimize that discomfort.

PSA TEST FOR PROSTATE CANCER

Q. *I recently read about a blood test for prostate cancer called PSA. How does this test work, and is it effective?*

A. Prostate-specific antigen, or PSA, is a protein made in the prostate gland and released into the bloodstream. The PSA blood test can indeed detect early prostate cancer. But it's often hard to tell whether an elevated reading signals cancer or merely benign enlargement of the prostate gland. Now researchers have found that repeating the PSA test each year can help physicians make that distinction.

Researchers at Johns Hopkins University found that PSA levels remain quite stable (below the "normal" limit of 4.0 micrograms per liter) in healthy men from year to year. In men with a noncancerous enlarged prostate, those levels rise only slightly each year. But cancer causes PSA scores to rise much faster.

The researchers concluded that even if the PSA level remains in the "normal" range, a jump of more than 0.75 microgram in one year is strong evidence of prostate cancer. Since a rapidly rising PSA level could signal a quick-growing tumor, an annual test might also help physicians determine whether immediate treatment is necessary.

We recommend that men age 50 and older (and African-American men age 45 and older) have the PSA test as well as a digital rectal exam every year.

HIGH PSA AND PROSTATE CANCER

Q. *My doctor ordered a PSA blood test for prostate cancer during a routine physical exam last fall. The results showed a score of 28, so he ordered a biopsy; it revealed no sign of cancer. I've since had another PSA test, which came out just as high. What, if anything, should I do about it?*

A. Talk to your doctor about having another biopsy—soon. A PSA (prostate-specific antigen) score above 10 indicates a strong probability of prostate cancer. The repeat biopsy should be guided by rectal ultrasound, which can help identify any suspicious areas in the prostate.

PROSTATE STONES

Q. *I have been diagnosed as having prostate stones. I'm worried that they might increase my chances of getting cancer. Will I pass these stones as kidney stones are sometimes passed?*

A. There's nothing to fear about so-called prostate stones. They're actually just tiny calcium deposits that form where the gland was inflamed at one time. Those "stones" can't be passed, and they don't lead to cancer.

PROSTATECTOMY AND INFERTILITY

Q. *You recently said that after surgery for an enlarged prostate, virtually all men become infertile due to "retrograde ejaculation," in which semen travels up into the bladder. Aren't there ways to isolate semen from the urine for artificial insemination?*

A. Yes. But the reliability of those techniques varies from person to person, depending on the viability of the sperm. Men who want to father a child after prostate surgery may also want to consider storing sperm at a sperm bank before the operation. However, that's not a sure bet either, since the freezing and thawing make sperm less vigorous.

IMPOTENCE AND BLOOD-PRESSURE DRUGS

Q. *The medication I take for high blood pressure is making me impotent. Is there a drug that can control my blood pressure without affecting my sex life?*

A. All of the widely used types of blood-pressure drugs have been associated in varying degrees with impotence. However, two classes of antihypertensive drugs may be less likely to cause impotence. One is a group known as ACE inhibitors, such as captopril (*Capoten*), enalapril (*Vasotec*), and lisinopril (*Prinivil, fosinopril*). The other group, called calcium-channel blockers, includes such drugs as diltiazem (*Cardizem*), nicardipine (*Cardene*), nifedipine (*Procardia*), and verapamil (*Calan, Isoptin*). If your current medication can be safely changed to one of those without compromising blood-pressure control, switching may solve your problem. If not, your physician might consider prescribing the impotence drug sildenafil, better known by its brand name, *Viagra*.

IMPOTENCE AND HORMONES

Q. *Six years ago, at age 65, I became impotent and had little sexual desire. Although my testosterone level was normal, I responded to hormone injections. However, my doctor refused to continue them for fear of stimulating latent prostate cancer cells. Now one prominent urologist is offering testosterone, while another says I would be "crazy" to take it. What's the story?*

A. The concern that testosterone may stimulate prostate cancer is reasonable. It's based on animal studies, the fact that testosterone accelerates prostate cancer growth, and the observation that prostatic cancer cells are present in a large percentage of aging men.

Moreover, there is no good clinical evidence that testosterone injections can improve potency in men with normal testosterone levels. Your positive reaction to the hormone may have been a placebo effect—a psychological response to taking medication. Other drugs are now available and worth discussing with your doctor: alprostadil *(Muse)* in the form of a pellet placed in the urethral opening or the oral drug sildenafil *(Viagra)*.

ADVICE GETS A "C"

Q. *Three years ago I underwent prostate surgery. Since then, on the advice of my urologist, I have been taking 500 milligrams of vitamin C twice a day to help prevent infection. Can you comment on this?*

A. The dose of vitamin C you're taking may make your urine somewhat acidic, but you can't count on it to inhibit bacterial growth. Nevertheless, you probably don't need to worry about infection. That risk presumably ended three years ago when the prostate surgery relieved your urinary obstruction.

PEYRONIE'S DISEASE

Q. *What can you tell me about Peyronie's disease?*

A. Peyronie's disease is a common disorder in which the penis becomes curved and distorted, especially when erect. The cause is unknown.

Local injections of steroids or calcium-channel blockers are sometimes successful. In carefully selected patients, surgery can sometimes be effective. It shouldn't be ruled out simply because of age. An experienced surgeon is necessary because of the possibility that surgery may create more scar tissue. When Peyronie's disease is combined with erectile dysfunction, the standard treatment is a penile implant. The recovery time for either procedure is about two weeks. Ask your doctor to refer you to a urologist experienced in treating this disease, or check the directory of the American Board of Medical Specialties, available at many libraries, for a list of board-certified specialists in your area.

Neurological problems

ARM NUMBNESS

Q. *I frequently have altered sensation and temperature perception in my right hand and arm. And one or both arms are often numb when I wake. What's the problem?*

A. Numbness or tingling in an arm during sleep is usually caused by pressure on a nerve, not poor circulation as is commonly believed. When one arm is affected, the pressure is often caused by a favorite sleeping position—for example, tucking your hand under your head or pillow. In that case, the numbness would disappear within a minute or two after you relieve the pressure. However, if the problem strikes both of your arms or either one during waking hours, you should be evaluated by a physician for other possible disorders, including carpal tunnel syndrome, disk disease of the neck or arthritis of the neck, and thoracic outlet obstruction syndrome.

HAND TREMOR

Q. *I've had a slight tremor in my hands for the past two or three years. In recent months it seems to have become more pronounced. Is there anything that can alleviate this condition?*

A. Yes, but the specific treatment depends on the underlying cause. Among the many causes for tremor: an overactive thyroid gland, Parkinson's disease, side effects of medications, too much caffeine, or anxiety.

Tremor can also run in families. The tremor should be evaluated by your physician, who may refer you to a neurologist for further investigation. More often than not, an appropriate medication can produce significant relief.

SCIATICA AND NUMB TOES

Q. *Last year I had sciatica from my back down to my right leg. The pain cleared up but left me with a kind of numbness in three toes (big toe and adjacent two) that I can't seem to shake. What can I do about this?*

A. Your numbness probably stems from some chronic irritation of the sciatic nerve root as it leaves the spinal cord. This may be caused by a herniated, or "slipped," disk, a disk fragment, or a bone spur. Unfortunately, the longer the numbness lasts, the less likely it is to disappear. A consultation with a neurologist would be advisable.

SLAPPING GAIT

Q. *What are the cause and treatment of "slap foot," which makes the front of the foot slap down noisily when walking?*

A. Slap foot, or what doctors call a slapping gait, results when something goes wrong with the nerves controlling the muscles in front of the lower leg. The weakened muscles can't lift the forefoot, which hits the ground before the heel. The problem could be caused by a bulging or herniated intervertebral disk or a bone spur pressing on the spinal cord. It could also be caused by a damaged or inflamed nerve supplying the front part of the leg. Treatment depends on identifying the cause. If no treatment is effective, a brace can be helpful.

TREATING A TREMOR

Q. *Are there any vitamins, minerals, or specific foods that might help the condition known as "benign essential tremor"?*

A. The medical term "essential" is often applied to conditions for which the cause is not known, and that unfortunately is the case with this troublesome neurological ailment. It sometimes runs in families, so there may be a genetic component. Unfortunately, there is no evidence that any nutritional therapy will improve this trembling of the hands, face, or voice. Small quantities of alcohol may temporarily suppress it, and beta-blocker drugs (such as propranolol or nadolol) frequently help. The anticonvulsant primidone *(Mysoline)* is also effective in some patients. In addition, one study with a small number of patients found about half responded well to a drug called methazolamide *(Neptazane)*, also used for glaucoma. However, those medications help the tremor only as long as they're being used. It may be more helpful to minimize intake of substances that can worsen tremors, such as caffeine, certain drugs for asthma, and oral decongestants.

Nose, mouth, and throat disorders

LOSS OF TASTE AND SMELL

Q. *At the age of 54, I seem to be losing my sense of taste and smell. What might be causing this?*

A. Like hearing and vision, taste and smell tend to deteriorate with age. In addition, various illnesses and injuries can damage the nerves connecting the sense organs to the brain. Loss of smell, for example, can be caused by nasal or sinus infections, nasal polyps, meningitis, or brain tumors. Loss of smell can affect taste. So can allergies, tongue injuries, stroke, or tumors. You should consult your physician to rule out possible underlying disorders.

SENSORY SHUTDOWN

Q. *My sense of smell has gradually deteriorated to the point that even pungent odors such as skunk spray don't register. I'm 35 years old and in excellent health with the exception of asthma, for which I take allergy injections, a steroid nasal spray, and other medications. Why am I losing my sense of smell?*

A. Two factors may be to blame. Your nasal passages may be sufficiently swollen from allergy-related causes, including nasal polyps, to limit your ability to detect odors. In addition, long-term use of a nasal spray could affect the smell receptors in your nasal membranes. A consultation with an otorhino-laryngologist (ear, nose, and throat specialist) may help.

BAD TASTE

Q. *I often notice a metallic taste in my mouth. What causes this and what can I do about it?*

A. Possible causes of your "dysgeusia," or distorted taste, range from allergies and nasal polyps to a prior head trauma or exposure to chemicals. It can also be a side effect of certain medications, particularly the antibiotics metronidazole (*Flagyl*), clarithromycin (*Biaxin*), or tetracycline. Sometimes metal fillings in your teeth may be the reason. Most often, however, no cause can be found.

In that case, there's nothing to do but wait it out. The sensation may last for years before it mysteriously disappears.

NAY TO NOSE SURGERY?

Q. *How necessary is surgery for a deviated septum? I believe this common operation corrects a birth defect and question its value on my 56-year-old nose.*

A. Most people are born with a straight septum, the cartilage-and-bone partition inside the nose. While some septal deviations are hereditary, many people incur slight deviations from minor childhood mishaps. Frequently, nasal congestion blamed on a deviated septum is caused by allergies, air pollution, pregnancy, or certain drugs. Short-term use of decongestants can usually clear the blocked airways.

When the deviation is severe and causes chronic breathing difficulty, repeated sinus infections, or chronic postnasal drip, removal of the obstructing portion of the septum can often provide permanent relief. However, a decision for surgery may be based on inadequate evidence of airway obstruction. So a second opinion should always be sought.

PROBLEMS WITH NASAL POLYPS

Q. *I have a nasal polyp that flares up each year for about a month and causes unbearable headaches. I had one removed surgically three years ago, but now the problem has recurred. Steroid nasal sprays seem to help, but I'm worried about using them. Are there any safer treatments?*

A. It's probably safe to continue with the sprays, especially for just one month a year. Very little of the steroid gets absorbed into the blood. A nasal polyp is actually swollen sinus tissue that protrudes into the nasal cavity. Polyps occur singly or in grapelike clusters. Since they're often caused by allergies, polyps can be treated the way allergies are—with antihistamines, decongestants, corticosteroid sprays, or even allergy shots. Alternatively, polyps can be removed surgically under local anesthesia. But as you can attest, additional ones can eventually appear.

RECURRENT SINUS INFECTIONS

Q. *What can I do about recurrent sinus infections? They clear up temporarily after antibiotics, but return in a couple of months. My doctor says X-rays show thickening in my sinuses.*

A. That thickening is due to chronic inflammation of the sinus lining. And an inflamed lining secretes excessive amounts of mucus, which predisposes you to yet another infection. You may need aggressive treatment with longer courses of antibiotics to break the cycle. Failing that, you should be evaluated by an otorhinolaryngologist (ear, nose, and throat specialist) for possible surgery to permit better drainage.

POSTNASAL DRIP

Q. *I suffer from postnasal drip, which constantly fills my throat with phlegm. What can I do about it?*

A. Probably not much. Postnasal drip is typically caused by air pollution, allergies, or infections. The irritated membranes in your nose and sinuses thicken and produce too much mucus. When the condition becomes chronic, it's often difficult to tell what caused it. And it's seldom cured.

Side effects from the standard medications used for postnasal drip—antibiotics, antihistamines, and decongestants—often outweigh their meager benefits. If you should try those drugs and they don't work, see an otorhinolaryngologist (ear, nose, and throat specialist). Once cysts, polyps, and tumors have been ruled out, either a corticosteroid nasal spray or cortisone injections into the nasal membranes may help.

NOSEBLEEDS

Q. *I've had allergies since I was a child. Four years ago, I had an operation for a broken nose. Now my nose bleeds if I happen to rub it—even only gently. Why?*

A. The problem probably has nothing to do with your broken nose or operation. But it may be related to your allergies—or, more precisely, your allergy medications. Antihistamines and decongestants can dry the mucous lining of the nasal passages. Rubbing, scratching, or other trauma can easily cause bleeding in a dry nose. To lessen drying, minimize your use of those medications and keep your environment comfortably humidified.

NONINHALED TOBACCO PRODUCTS

Q. *Health reports often warn about the dangers of cigarette smoking. What are the risks of using noninhaled tobacco products such as pipes, cigars, and chewing tobacco?*

A. The fact is that some pipe and cigar smokers do inhale, even unconsciously. Aside from the known risks of inhaled smoke, the main danger is cancer of the mouth, tongue and throat. The risk is greater in people who also drink a lot of alcohol. In addition, nicotine is easily absorbed through the lining of the mouth, and that increases the risk of coronary heart disease.

PHARYNGITIS DEMYSTIFIED

Q. *I've seen references to "pharyngitis" and haven't been able to figure out what it is. My dictionary says it's inflammation of the pharynx, which is "the part of the vertebrate alimentary canal between the cavity of the mouth and the esophagus." Please translate.*

A. It's a sore throat.

THRUSH

Q. *A few months ago I developed "thrush"—whitish patches on my tongue and on the back of my throat—after a six-day course of intravenous antibiotics. The antibiotics apparently killed the normal protective bacteria in my mouth, allowing the thrush to develop. Now I'm concerned about my intestinal bacteria as well. So I've been taking L. acidophilus and bifidus supplements to reestablish those bacteria. Is that the right thing to do?*

A. No. The bacterial imbalance that follows use of antibiotics may indeed allow other bacteria or fungi to take hold. Those include the candida that cause thrush. But the "intestinal flora" supplements you mention have never been shown to help prevent or treat that imbalance. You should treat the candida with an effective antifungal medicine, such as oral nystatin (*Mycostatin*). The usual bacterial population will return to your mouth and intestinal tract on its own.

AGING: HARD TO SWALLOW

Q. *Older people often seem to choke on food, cough a lot while eating, or swallow "the wrong way." What are the cause and treatment for those reflexes?*

A. As people age, the muscles in the back of the throat and upper esophagus, which are responsible for swallowing, often become less well coordinated. Most older people don't notice that gradual change unless it's compounded by other factors—for instance, poor chewing due to problems with teeth or dentures, or eating or drinking too rapidly.

To help prevent choking, try to chew food well, swallow carefully, and eat in an upright position. If you wear dentures, make sure they fit properly.

SWALLOWING DIFFICULTIES

Q. *I have esophageal achalasia, which makes swallowing extremely difficult. Other than eating finely chopped food or chewing food thoroughly, is surgery the only way to correct my problem?*

A. No. Only about one out of four patients eventually requires surgery. In achalasia, the muscular ring, or sphincter, between the esophagus and the stomach fails to open adequately when you swallow. Treatment depends on the severity of the condition, which is determined by taking X-rays and examining the esophagus through an endoscope, a flexible lighted tube. (Since achalasia may increase the risk of esophageal cancer, endoscopy checks for that possibility as well.)

There are two nonsurgical alternatives. Medications such as nifedipine (*Procardia*) may relax the sphincter. If not, a special instrument can be passed down the throat to widen the sphincter by splitting the constricting muscle fibers.

RASH IN THE MOUTH

Q. *What can you tell me about oral lichen planus? Is there a treatment?*

A. Lichen planus is a common disease that appears in the mouth, on the skin, or both. The oral version often shows up as a lacelike network of white lines located on the inside of the cheeks. The disease can also take the form of open sores on the gums, tongue, palate, floor of the mouth, or lips. Those sores can cause bleeding and pain and hamper proper dental care. At its worst, the inflammation can even interfere with eating, swallowing, and speaking. People in their 40s and 50s are more prone to lichen planus than other age groups, and the cause has never been identified.

Treatment for oral lichen planus depends on the severity of the disease. If you have only the white lacy lines, no treatment may be necessary, since those lines cause no other symptoms. For those who have sores, treatment frequently consists of a corticosteroid paste *(Kenalog)* or gel *(Lidex, Temovate)*. Though treatment is often effective at promoting healing, the disease can often recur over several years. The antifungal oral rinse nystatin *(Mycostatin, Nilstat, Nystex)* is often prescribed along with corticosteroids, since individuals who have lichen planus are at increased risk of oral yeast infections, and corticosteroids boost that risk even further.

Severe lichen planus can sometimes be the first sign of an undiagnosed case of hepatitis C, so individuals with severe symptoms should also be screened for the hepatitis C virus. Patients with oral lichen planus are at higher risk of squamous-cell carcinoma and should have their mouths checked for cancer at least once a year.

COATED TONGUE

Q. *Recently I noticed a white film on my tongue that I can't seem to remove by brushing. Any suggestions?*

A. First, try to track down the cause of your coated tongue. Sometimes it's a change in diet. If so, try eliminating the suspected offender, and see if the coating disappears. Ask your physician whether the culprit could be a yeast infection or medication you have taken—particularly antibiotics and medications that dry the mouth, such as antihistamines.

When the cause can't be determined or corrected, brushing the tongue with a soft-bristle toothbrush does help some people. Since that didn't help you, you might simply try drinking more fluids. In time, the condition will probably disappear on its own.

EAT AND RUN

Q. *Why does my nose run while I'm eating or after I eat? It happens with all types of foods, and mainly after dinner.*

A. You're experiencing what's called prandial rhinorrhea, meaning—sure enough—the free discharge of a thin nasal mucus, associated with a meal. Eating activates the autonomic nervous system, which releases the chemical acetylcholine. That in turn gets the body's juices flowing, including saliva and stomach acid as well as nasal mucus and sometimes tears. The degree of reaction varies widely. Usually, the spicier the meal, the greater the reaction.

If your problem is severe, try taking an antihistamine or a decongestant before you eat. If that doesn't do the trick, consult your physician.

Pain medications

ASPIRIN, IBUPROFEN, AND CLOTTING

Q. *Is there any difference between aspirin and ibuprofen in their tendency to inhibit the blood-clotting action of platelets?*

A. Yes—though it's a difference in degree. A daily dose of three 200-milligram ibuprofen tablets (*Advil, Motrin-IB*) can inhibit platelet function for about 24 hours. It takes only about one-third of a single 325-milligram aspirin tablet to inhibit platelets for up to a week. While people with bleeding

disorders must avoid aspirin, they may be able to use ibuprofen under a doctor's supervision.

ASPIRIN AND HEARING

Q. *I frequently take aspirin and have lately begun to wonder if it affects my hearing. Can it?*

A. Yes. Hearing loss and tinnitus (ringing in the ears) have been recognized for more than a century as signs of aspirin toxicity. When those problems are caused by too much aspirin, both problems disappear on reducing the aspirin dosage. If either problem persists, check with your physician.

ASPIRIN GONE BAD

Q. *I have always heard that you should discard aspirin when it begins to smell like vinegar. The last bottle I bought has an expiration date of two years from now, but it already has that vinegary odor. Is such aspirin harmful?*

A. No, just less effective. The odor indicates that the drug is breaking down into its constituent parts. That happens gradually but begins as soon as you first open the bottle. Even fresh aspirin has some vinegary smell. But if the odor is very strong in a previously unopened bottle, replace it. To slow the decomposition, store aspirin in a cool, dry place (not the bathroom) and keep the cap tightly closed.

HOW MUCH ASPIRIN?

Q. *My neurologist has prescribed a daily 81-milligram aspirin tablet to prevent stroke. Would a higher dose be more effective?*

A. It's unlikely but not certain. While some studies demonstrating protection against stroke have used as much as 1,800 milligrams of aspirin a day, none has shown any added benefit over daily doses as low as 50 to 100 milligrams. The Food and Drug Administration recently endorsed a range of 50 milligrams to no more than 325 milligrams (the amount in an ordinary, regular-strength aspirin tablet) for people who are at risk for a thrombotic (clot-related) stroke *or* a heart attack. The lower the dose, the lower the chance of side effects, which can include heartburn and stomach bleeding. Because of the possible adverse effects, it's essential to consult a physician before starting an aspirin regimen—whatever the dose.

ASPIRIN AND HERBAL BLOOD THINNERS

Q. *I know that taking a baby aspirin each day can help prevent blood clots in the arteries. I've also heard many people recommend garlic capsules, ginger tea, and ginkgo biloba for that purpose. Which strategy is better? Or would it be OK to take both aspirin and the herbs?*

A. The three herbs you mention do appear to have some anticlotting effect, but only aspirin has been shown to help reduce the risk of heart attack and clot-related stroke. Moreover, because aspirin is such a potent blood-thinner, even a low-dose "baby" aspirin might interact with any of those herbs and pose a possible risk of bleeding problems.

PAIN IN THE NECK

Q. *When I walk uphill rapidly, I get a slight pain in the left side of my neck. My doctor ordered a treadmill test, which showed nothing abnormal. I'm 60 years old. What could the pain be?*

A. There are two main possibilities: One is simple arthritic or muscular pain. If holding your head in certain positions sparks the pain, the problem might well be musculoskeletal.

Or it could be an atypical form of angina pectoris, a symptom of insufficient blood circulation to the heart. The pain is usually centered in the chest but may sometimes be felt only in the neck.

If physical exertion triggers the pain, coronary heart disease must be suspected. That's why your doctor tested you on a treadmill—to see whether the exercise would either provoke the pain or reveal evidence of inadequate circulation on an electrocardiogram.

Unfortunately, a normal result on a standard treadmill stress test does not necessarily exclude coronary disease. To rule that out more definitively, you may need a nuclear stress test, in which a radioactive chemical is injected into the bloodstream during exercise and the heart is scanned by a radiation detector. If the nuclear test shows an abnormality, then angiography *may* be necessary.

TRIGEMINAL NEURALGIA

Q. *I have trigeminal neuralgia, which causes excruciating pain on one side of my face. The drug* Tegretol *eliminates the pain but leaves me confused, drowsy, and depressed. Is there any alternative treatment?*

A. To start with, your physician may be able to reduce your dosage of carbamazepine (*Tegretol*) without compromising the drug's effectiveness. If that doesn't work, your physician might try other drugs, such as phenytoin (*Dilantin*) or amitriptyline (*Elavil*).

It's also possible to deaden the particular nerve that's causing the pain, using alcohol or glycerol injections, nerve blocks, radio frequency waves through the skin, or surgery. However, those procedures can leave part of your face permanently numb.

FELDENE SIDE EFFECTS

Q. *I have a gnawing ache in my left thigh, diagnosed as pressure on a nerve from a bulging vertebral disk. My doctor prescribed* Feldene, *which helps. But will I have trouble with side effects if I keep using it?*

A. Perhaps. About 30 percent of patients who take piroxicam (*Feldene*) report adverse effects—most often gastrointestinal complaints, such as upset stomach, nausea, constipation, diarrhea, or flatulence. Such problems force about 5 percent of users to stop taking the drug.

Like aspirin, piroxicam and all other nonsteroidal antiinflammatory drugs (such as fenoprofen, ibuprofen, and naproxen) can cause slight blood loss in the stool, although it may not be readily visible. Over a period of months, this can cause anemia. A physician should check your blood count every two or three months. People who bleed easily, take anticoagulants, or are sensitive to aspirin should avoid piroxicam.

Respiratory infections

ANTIBIOTICS FOR A BAD COLD

Q. *I've had two particularly bad colds over the past year. Both times, my doctor prescribed antibiotics. I thought that a cold is a viral infection and that antibiotics aren't effective against viruses. Why the antibiotics?*

A. That depends. Antibiotics indeed won't do anything for a viral infection such as the common cold. But sometimes a cold virus leads to a bacterial infection in the sinus or bronchial airways, which does require antibiotics.

A physician typically makes that decision by looking for signs of bacterial infection. Sinus infections can produce a thick, yellow discharge from the nose, tenderness or pain just above or below the eyes, and perhaps a slight fever. Bronchial infections can also cause fever as well as a cough that brings up greenish yellow sputum or even some blood.

If you have none of those symptoms, you probably shouldn't take antibiotics. The drugs can cause such side effects as nausea, diarrhea, and rashes. They can also kill off the body's own protective bacteria, allowing fungal infections to grow.

WHERE THERE'S SMOKE

Q. *A year or so ago I was diagnosed as having a bronchial infection caused by* Hemophilus influenza *bacteria. Despite having taken three or four antibiotics, I still have a very productive cough. Could the fact that I smoke cigarettes be hampering my recovery?*

A. Very likely. Not only do smokers experience more respiratory infections than nonsmokers do, but they also are likely to have more difficulty recovering. Smoking destroys cilia, the tiny filaments that help to move infected mucus up and out of the lungs. And the ability of the lungs to repair tissue damage is impaired by years of smoking.

Skin care

SCRATCHING AN ITCH

Q. *For months I've been suffering from an annoying itch. It starts in one spot, I scratch it, and it turns red and bumpy. Then it disappears and starts up again somewhere else. I've been taking an antihistamine, which helps, but I'm worried. What's wrong with me?*

A. The red, bumpy rashes you describe are probably the result of scratching, not the cause of the itch. Unexplained generalized itching, called pruritus, has several possible causes. Older people often itch in the winter because their skin becomes drier. Using water-soluble lubricating oils, bathing less frequently, and running a room humidifier may help. Certain systemic diseases, such as diabetes, liver disease, and some forms of cancer, can also cause itching. These can easily be excluded by appropriate tests. If the cause is unknown, antihistamines, such as hydroxyzine (*Atarax, Vistaril*), can help.

ITCHING ALL OVER

Q. *For the past two years, I've itched from my scalp to the soles of my feet, including the palms of my hands, my ears, and my eyes. There is no rash. At night the itching is accompanied by muscular spasms in my legs and a burning sensation. Please help.*

A. Persistent itching can be caused by allergies to food or medications, and by skin disorders such as scabies (which don't always have visible signs). The burning sensation you've experienced could be a sign of nerve inflammation. A physical exam is needed to find the cause for your itching. If your physician can find no treatable cause, he or she may recommend an oral antihistamine such as hydroxyzine (*Atarax, Vistaril*) to relieve the symptoms.

ECZEMA

Q. *I have eczema on my hands and feet—blisters, itching, peeling, cracking, and bleeding—that gets worse in the winter. What can I do about it?*

A. Since scratching the skin prolongs the problem, avoid any irritant, such as wool, synthetic fibers, animal fur, or soap.

Any of them might set off the itch-scratch cycle. To soothe your skin, keep it well lubricated with bland lotions. Over-the-counter hydrocortisone creams (*CaldeCORT, Cortaid*) may also help, but when used over a long period of time, they can thin the skin. This can reduce the skin's effectiveness as a protective barrier and make it more vulnerable to trauma. Avoid preparations that contain anesthetics, antihistamines, or other chemicals alleged to relieve itching; they may cause allergic reactions when applied to inflamed skin.

HARRIED BY HIVES

Q. *About a week ago I suddenly developed hives—blistery blotches on my skin that seem to appear and disappear within a short time. Why would hives wait until I was 67 years old before appearing? What could be causing them?*

A. Hives can show up at any age. Unfortunately, their cause remains a mystery close to 70 percent of the time. Allergies to food, food additives, medication, or other ingested substances probably account for most cases. If the hives recur frequently, keeping a diary of your food and medication might provide a clue to the specific agent. Cold, heat, and even physical pressure can give some people hives as well.

Anxiety and emotional upset are overrated as a cause of hives but can provoke an occasional outbreak. While you're searching for an explanation for your case, antihistamines can relieve the discomfort. Occasionally, temporary use of a prescription steroid medication may be necessary.

DRY-LIP DISTRESS

Q. *I am troubled by very dry lips for which no cause has been found. Following my doctor's advice, I use cortisone cream and special lipsticks, but the condition persists. I have also tried all kinds of vitamins, to no avail. Any further advice?*

A. Extremely dry lips, known as cheilitis, can sometimes be traced to a contact allergy (to lipsticks, lip salves, mouthwash, or toothpaste), to nighttime drooling or frequent lip licking or, rarely, to a deficiency of iron or vitamin B_2 (riboflavin). Often, however, the cause remains obscure. Systematically avoiding each suspect product—one at a time—may uncover the one responsible. Also steer clear of oral medications containing antihistamines, which tend to dry the mucous membranes of the mouth. To moisten and protect your lips, use a nonirritating product such as petroleum jelly (*Vaseline*), and apply a lip balm containing a sunblock when outdoors.

COLD SORES AND SHINGLES

Q. *I have recurring cold sores on my mouth and chin. I've heard that the herpes simplex virus that causes them is related to the virus that causes shingles. Does that mean I'm more likely to get shingles eventually?*

A. No. Shingles, also known as herpes zoster, is caused by the varicella zoster virus, the same virus that causes chicken pox. Although the skin lesions of the herpes simplex virus are similar to those caused by the varicella zoster virus, the two viruses are still quite distinct. It's not known why the varicella zoster virus resurfaces years later as shingles in up to 20 percent of people who have had chicken pox—but it's not because they have cold sores.

SHINGLES: THE AFTEREFFECTS

Q. *About a year ago, my wife contracted a severe case of shingles. Although the rash is gone now, the severe pain persists. Her doctors have prescribed only pain-relief pills. Is there a permanent cure?*

A. The pain that remains after an attack of shingles is known as postherpetic neuralgia, and it is notoriously hard to vanquish. Some drugs have proved helpful, but not for all people. They include capsaicin (often sold as *Zostrix*), a topical medication; amitriptyline (*Elavil*), an antidepressant; phenytoin (*Dilantin*) and carbamazepine (*Tegretol*), both anticonvulsants; and injections of corticosteroids. In other people, only time brings relief; the pain can last for months or years.

Some dermatologists now prescribe oral cortisone, taken for three weeks after shingles first appears, to prevent the pain that persists after an attack. But the efficacy of this particular treatment remains unproven.

ROSACEA

Q. *I have rosacea, mostly on my cheeks. What can I do about it?*

A. In some people, avoiding hot or spicy foods, hot beverages, and alcohol will minimize this chronic blood-vessel inflammation, which appears as redness or pustules on the cheeks, nose, chin, forehead, or eyelids. If those measures don't help, your physician can prescribe oral or topical antibiotics that will control the condition. If that doesn't work, a doctor might prescribe metronidazole gel *(MetroGel)* for a particularly stubborn case. But avoid hydrocortisone cream; long-term use can cause changes that resemble rosacea itself.

SKIN GROWTHS

Q. *I have a bad case of seborrheic keratoses—grayish, molelike growths all over my torso. They're not painful, but they are unsightly. What should I do?*

A. Seborrheic keratoses don't become cancerous, so they're purely a cosmetic matter. A dermatologist could remove them easily, since the soft growths don't adhere strongly to the skin. Most dermatologists simply freeze the skin to numb it and then scrape the growths off with a curette (a rounded cutting instrument). If necessary, an electric current first destroys the growths.

The procedure produces minimal bleeding and the wounds heal without scarring. However, you may be uncomfortable while you're healing, and it could cost several hundred dollars to have the more pervasive growths removed.

CRACKED HEELS

Q. *Winter or summer, the skin on my heels cracks and splits, sometimes to the point of bleeding. What causes this problem and how can I rid myself of it?*

A. First see your physician to check for fungus infection or psoriasis. If those are ruled out, your heels are probably cracking because the skin is too dry. A common treatment involves "moisture trapping"—tap-water baths followed by immediate application of a nonirritating agent such as mineral oil or petroleum jelly before putting on socks and shoes. Other creams and lotions containing water or fragrances may exacerbate the problem, so it's best to avoid them.

REMOVING BLACKHEADS

Q. *What's the safest, most effective way to remove blackheads on the nose or elsewhere on the face?*

A. If your blackheads are associated with facial acne, seek professional help because of the possibility of infection. For the occasional blackhead, first wash your face (and hands) with soap and warm water, then press down the skin around the blackhead to extrude the oxidized matter plugging the pore. Contrary to myth, this practice does no harm.

TETRACYCLINE FOR ACNE

Q. *I've been taking tetracycline for several years to treat my adult acne. Are there any side effects?*

A. Usually only minor ones. Tetracycline and other antibiotics help suppress acne-promoting bacteria in the skin's oil glands. Doctors often prescribe long-term tetracycline treatment for moderately severe acne. After a few weeks at full dosage, the dose is reduced to the smallest amount that will control the problem. Years of experience—thousands of patients and millions of prescriptions—have shown that side effects are usually mild and disappear when the drug is discontinued. Among the most common ones are diarrhea, stomach cramps, and vaginal yeast infections. In some people, tetracycline makes the skin more sensitive to ultraviolet radiation—and more susceptible to severe sunburn. Pregnant or breast-feeding women should avoid tetracycline; it may discolor the teeth of the fetus or newborn infant and slow the growth of the infant's teeth and bones.

If you are taking any other drugs along with tetracycline, you should tell your doctor, since some drugs may decrease the effect of tetracycline. Conversely, if you are taking oral contraceptives containing estrogen along with tetracycline, the tetracycline may decrease the effect of the birth-control pills and thus increase the possibility of unwanted pregnancy.

ACNE SCARS IN MIDDLE AGE

Q. *I'm in my early forties. Because of teenage acne, my complexion is severely pitted and pockmarked. Is there any treatment or procedure to relieve this condition?*

A. A procedure called dermabrasion, in which the skin is literally sanded down, can make scars less obvious and improve overall appearance. This procedure is usually performed under local anesthesia, and can be done by a dermatologist or plastic surgeon on an outpatient basis. After dermabrasion, the skin remains uncomfortably raw for 10 to 14 days; redness may linger for as long as several months.

CYSTS ON THE SCALP

Q. *My brother and I suffer from sebaceous cysts on the scalp. As the cysts enlarge, they itch and hurt when bumped. We've had several of them removed, but they're back in the same places within a few years. Is there any way to get rid of these growths permanently?*

A. When located in the scalp, a skin cyst (properly called a pilar cyst or wen) generally originates with a hair follicle. Elsewhere on the body, a skin cyst (or epidermoid cyst) usually originates with a sebaceous gland duct. Both kinds are benign, saclike swellings beneath the surface of the skin.

Most skin cysts don't need to be removed unless they become infected, painful, or cosmetically unacceptable. If a surgeon removes an entire cyst intact, it won't reform, but more cysts can occur elsewhere. Indeed, many people who tend to form skin cysts have multiple occurrences.

ELECTROLYSIS AND MOLES

Q. *I've been going for electrolysis to remove the hairs that grow from several moles on my face. One dermatologist told me it's dangerous to have electrolysis on mole hairs. Another said it's perfectly safe. Who's right?*

A. The one who said it's safe. Some people believe that removing hairs or otherwise disturbing a mole might trigger cancerous changes. However, there's no evidence to support that notion.

FAREWELL TO KELOID SCARS

Q. *I've had keloids on my chest for 25 years and they seem to get thicker and more itchy each day. I've had them removed by both conventional and laser surgery and injected with cortisone, but they always come back. Can anything more be done?*

A. Keloids are thick, raised, ropy scars that can occur after a surgical procedure or accidental laceration. The tendency to develop keloids appears to be hereditary. In certain people—particularly African-Americans, Asians, and Hispanics—recurrence is common and hard to avoid. Treatment depends on both the size and location of the keloid and includes injection with corticosteriods, surgical removal, laser therapy, cryosurgery, and others. As with any disorder that has multiple treatments, no one particular method is good for all patients.

It's best to remove the keloid and immediately inject the area with cortisone. Additional injections should be given at the first sign of itching, which foreshadows the keloid's reappearance. Within two years, most keloids treated this way are permanently banished. Keloids that aren't bothersome in comfort or appearance can be safely left alone.

NO CURE FOR VITILIGO

Q. *I have had vitiligo for more than 20 years. When I was first diagnosed, I was told there was no treatment for this condition. Is that still the case?*

A. Yes and no. There's still no cure for vitiligo, the patchy loss of skin pigmentation. But newer, more sophisticated skin dyes—hydroxyacetone, for example—can help to camouflage the whitish patches. Oral medications called psoralens can sometimes sensitize any remaining pigment cells to stimulation by ultraviolet light, helping to retard further loss of skin color. But this treatment may increase the risk of skin cancer and should be reserved for severe cases. Unfortunately, treatment with psoralens usually isn't effective in cases as long-standing as yours. Vitiligo patches can be especially vulnerable to sunburn, so the use of sunscreens is recommended.

DERMATITIS FROM HAIR DYE

Q. *Having dyed my hair for the past two years, I am now suffering the consequences—acute dermatitis. According to two dermatologists, the results could have been much worse. What happened?*

A. You seem to have developed a sensitivity to the chemical paraphenylenediamine, a component of many hair dyes. This can cause local swelling and blistering of the scalp. "Cross-sensitization" often occurs, which means that you may now experience a similar reaction to other dyes, certain anesthetics, and even to PABA (the active ingredient in some sunscreens). From now on, you would be wise to use hypoallergenic products whenever they are available.

PURPLE PEOPLE

Q. *When I was a Marine stationed in the tropics, jock itch was a common problem. The smiling medic would swab on gentian violet, and you'd walk away cured (on fire, but cured). Why don't I hear about that old standby anymore?*

A. Because few doctors use it anymore. Gentian violet (methylrosaniline) was a popular remedy for skin or vaginal problems caused by fungi or bacteria 20 to 30 years ago. It was even taken by mouth for intestinal worms. Gentian violet has been replaced by more effective drugs that don't turn you or your socks or underwear purple.

SPOTTING SKIN CANCER

Q. *Should a thorough inspection of the skin be part of a comprehensive physical examination?*

A. Yes. Each year about 1,000,000 new cases of skin cancer are diagnosed in the United States, and more than 9,000 people die from the disease. Total body examinations are crucial for early detection and treatment of both skin cancers and premalignant skin lesions. Removal of the lesions usually results in a complete cure, especially if they are detected at an early stage.

If your doctor fails to include a total body exam in your physical, ask for it. If you're at increased risk for skin cancer (because of previous cancerous lesions, family history, or fair complexion), you may want to consult a dermatologist for the exam.

TANNING LOTIONS AND PILLS

Q. *Are tanning lotions and tanning pills safe?*

A. Yes and no, respectively. The lotions usually contain dihydroxyacetone, or DHA. They can create an uneven, somewhat off-colored, orangy tan, but they're safe enough.

Tanning pills are not only unsafe, they're illegal. The FDA has approved canthaxanthin, the pills' active ingredient, only for use at very low levels to color some foods and drugs. Used in tanning pills, the dye turns the skin golden orange. It can also build up in the retina and liver, and cause skin reactions, itching, and abnormal liver function tests.

The FDA first warned against the use of such tanning pills in 1981. Since then, the agency has banned the products and seized them occasionally but has not been able to keep them off the market. The pills are still marketed through mail-order ads in newspapers and bodybuilding magazines. They're also sold at some health-food stores and tanning salons.

EASY BRUISING

Q. *I'm 75 years old and have purpura. What can I do about it?*

A. That depends on the cause. Purpura is a catchall term for bleeding into the skin, which creates purple bruises. Anything that affects the surface blood vessels or platelets (blood cells essential to clotting) can cause purpura. The most likely cause of your purpura is simply the loss, with age, of the protective skin tissue around those blood vessels. There's no treatment for the condition, although avoiding bumps or pressure on the skin may help.

However, you should see a physician to rule out more serious problems. Those include allergies and other reactions to drugs (including aspirin) and diseases affecting the platelets or bone marrow.

DISCOID LUPUS

Q. *My husband was recently told he might have discoid lupus, although lab tests were normal. Is this a dangerous disease?*

A. Not by itself. Discoid lupus erythematosus typically causes red, round, scaly rashes. It is, however, related to a more serious disease, systemic lupus erythematosus. Systemic lupus can affect just about every part of the body, including the kidneys and other vital organs.

A skin biopsy can identify discoid lupus; special blood tests are required to identify systemic lupus. Up to 20 percent of patients who have the discoid rash also have the systemic disease. If your husband has discoid lupus but blood tests do not detect systemic lupus, he has about a 95 percent chance of not developing the systemic disease.

A BATHROOM SUNBURN?

Q. *I use an infrared bulb to warm my bathroom. How much ultraviolet (UV) radiation is given off by those bulbs?*

A. The amount of UV radiation emitted by an infrared bulb is negligible—even less than that emitted by an ordinary bulb.

SPLIT FINGERNAILS

Q. *I'm concerned about my fingernails repeatedly splitting to the quick. What can I take to strengthen them and prevent splits?*

A. Nothing you ingest—including the oft-recommended gelatin and calcium—will strengthen your fingernails. Splitting is most often caused by a minor injury to the nail itself. The biggest culprit is water—more specifically, alternating periods of wetness and dryness. So avoid soaking your hands in water. The overuse of nail polish remover can also cause splitting. Other persistent nail deformities—ridging, pitting, and odd shapes—may reflect chronic diseases or a previous acute illness.

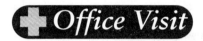

WHAT'S IN AN ITCH

"Let me tell you, Cassius, you yourself are much condemned to have an itching palm," declared Brutus during a feisty encounter with his coconspirator in Shakespeare's *Julius Caesar*. By indulging his corrupt impulses, Cassius earned the condemnation of his more honorable partner.

In life as in art, scratching a persistent itch, while pleasurable in the moment, can condemn you to greater discomfort in the long run. Far better to get to the root of the itch. There's often an underlying problem that can be corrected.

WHAT MAKES YOU ITCH?

The itch sensation travels the same nerve fibers that carry pain signals to the spinal cord and brain. Apparently, scratching brings relief by overwhelming the itch with an even stronger sensation.

When the cause of itching is not obvious, a physician may be tempted to diagnose a "nervous itch." But while emotional stress can aggravate itching, psychological factors are rarely the underlying cause. There's usually a medical explanation.

It's easiest to find the cause when itching is limited to one particular area of the body.

Itching feet or an itch in the groin area is usually due to fungal infection. A mild case may turn the skin reddish brown; in severe cases, the skin can crack, become raw, and even bleed. You can treat a mild infection with over-the-counter antifungal creams and powders, such as clotrimazole (*Lotrimin AF*) or miconazole (*Micatin*). Severe inflammation could indicate a bacterial infection on top of the fungal infection. In that case, an antifungal product could make the problem worse; see your doctor instead.

Anal itching can also be caused by fungal infections—as well as by hemorrhoids, skin fissures, sweating, worms, or poor anal hygiene. Each problem has its own treatment, ranging from careful cleansing to hydrocortisone cream.

Scabies, which can cause intense itching just about anywhere on the body, is caused by a microscopic mite that burrows under the skin. If you look closely, you'll see little ridges or dotted lines ending in tiny blisters. Treatment consists of using a pesticide-containing cream or lotion. Even after the mite has been successfully eradicated, though, the itch can persist for weeks.

WHEN SCRATCHING HURTS

Sometimes, localized itching can actually be caused by scratching. This condition, known as neurodermatitis, is not an actual nerve disorder but rather a vicious spiral of itching and repeated scratching that leads to gradual thickening and darkening of the skin; the area then itches more than ever. Neurodermatitis is seen most often on the nape or side of the neck, but can develop anywhere.

The only way to eliminate neurodermatitis is to break the itch-scratch cycle:

• Don't wear irritating fabrics such as wool, silk, or rough synthetics. Instead, try to wear absorbent, nonirritating materials next to the skin.

• To suppress the urge to scratch, apply an ice-cold compress.

• You might want to apply an over-the-counter hydrocortisone cream (*Cortaid*) and cover with a bandage. (But don't use such drugs for longer than two to three weeks, since they can thin the skin.)

• If itching makes it hard for you to fall asleep, try an over-the-counter antihistamine such as diphenhydramine (*Benadryl Allergy*). A simple over-the-counter pain reliever—such as aspirin, acetaminophen (*Tylenol*), or ibuprofen (*Advil*)—can also bring relief.

• Since many sufferers scratch when they're asleep, keep your fingernails short.

WHERE THERE'S A RASH

A widespread itchy rash indicates other problems. Sometimes, an allergic reaction to a certain food or medication will lead to a sudden bout of hives—a raised red rash that spreads over the body and itches like crazy. Although such a reaction usually occurs within just a few hours after ingesting the offending food or drug, it can take as long as a week to show up after a final dose of certain antibiotics, including penicillin. Many times, expert detective work is needed to track down the culprit.

In addition to things that you ingest, things that you touch can also make you itch. Contact dermatitis can be brought on by plants, cosmetics, chemicals, even rough clothing and harsh soaps or laundry detergents. Hours or possibly days after contact, a very itchy, red, blistery rash develops. Again, the trick is to identify and avoid the offending item.

Silvery, scaly patches are a sure sign of psoriasis. While the condition commonly occurs on the elbows or knees, it can also affect the entire body, including the scalp. The rash isn't always itchy, but it can be—very. Psoriasis usually clears temporarily in response to ultraviolet light, either from sunlight or a special lamp. If there are only small patches, a hydrocortisone cream can help. Or your doctor may prescribe a more potent corticosteroid cream.

ITCHING ALL OVER

When there's no sign of a rash, itching "all over" can be a symptom of an internal disorder. Such itching can signal diseases of the liver, kidneys, or thyroid gland. If lab tests detect such a disease, proper treatment can resolve the itch as well.

By far the most common cause of generalized itching without a noticeable rash is simply dry skin. As you age, your skin thins and oil glands produce less of a protective barrier on the skin surface. This leaves your skin more vulnerable to minor irritations. The problem is especially severe in wintertime, when humidity is low.

Fortunately, there are several ways you can protect your skin:

• To preserve your natural protective oils, take shorter and less frequent baths or showers, and use lukewarm water.

• Use a mild soap—one that's low in alkaline, such as *Dove* or *Neutrogena*. Apply the soap only to your face, armpits, genital and anal areas, and hands and feet.

• If you bathe rather than shower, add a little water-dispersible bath oil, such as *Alpha Keri*. (Be sure to use a rubber mat in the tub to avoid slipping.)

• Immediately after bathing, apply bath oil to your moist skin. Avoid alcohol-containing lotions, which dry out the skin.

• Don't air-dry after bathing; that tends to chap your skin. Pat dry with an absorbent towel.

• Use a room humidifier during winter.

• Keep room temperatures on the cool side, since warmth can worsen an itch.

• In cold weather, wear gloves and a scarf or ski mask to limit the evaporation of moisture from your hands and face.

• Use a mild laundry detergent that has no enzymes or perfumes. Rinse clothes well.

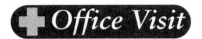

FINGERNAIL PROBLEMS: SERIOUS— OR JUST ANNOYING?

Several years ago, a 28-year-old high-school teacher came to see me about her deformed, pitted fingernails. She had already seen a dermatologist, who prescribed antifungal medication despite the absence of any evidence of a fungal infection. Not surprisingly, the treatment didn't help.

Besides bad nails, she also complained of aches and pains in several joints, especially in her fingers. When I examined her, I found red and silver scaly patches on both elbows—characteristic signs of the skin disorder psoriasis. That solved the mystery of her nail problem: Psoriasis is often accompanied by both nail pitting and arthritis pain.

Since fingernails sometimes provide clues to the presence of various disorders, physicians will often check the nails during a complete exam. (So remove any nail polish in advance!) In most cases, however, nail problems stem from ordinary wear and tear. Here I'll discuss both disease and damage.

DEFORMITY AND DISEASE

Nails often have bumps and other flaws that don't signal a problem. Vertical ridges become more common and usually more pronounced as people age. White lines and tiny white spots are common, too. The following unusual nail features, on the other hand, may indeed reflect disease:

• Deformities such as pitting, spooning (in which the nail curls upward), and separation of the nail from its bed can be caused by diseases as diverse as anemia and hypothyroidism, as well as psoriasis.

• Nail color, usually a healthy pink, can also indicate disease. Pale or whitish nails, for example, suggest anemia; bluish nails, due to insufficient oxygen in the blood, could mean poisoning, heart failure, or chronic lung trouble.

• Rounding and expansion of both the nails and the ends of the fingers, which may become clublike, can reflect a variety of serious conditions, ranging from lung cancer to inflammatory bowel disease.

• A horizontal furrow, or "Beau's line," can result from major surgery, heart attack, or other serious illness, which can slow nail growth abruptly. The line eventually grows out.

• Thick, distorted nails, especially on the toes, often indicate a fungal infection. While the condition can be painful, it's usually only a cosmetic concern. Oral antifungal drugs, such as itraconazole *(Sporanox)* and terbinafine *(Lamisil)*, can clear up most cases.

WEAR AND TEAR

Nail weakness is probably the most common fingernail problem. A number of diseases, such as an overactive thyroid and anemia, can make the nails brittle. Usually, though, nails weaken simply because they're subjected to so much everyday abuse.

Take water, for example, the most common cause of brittle nails. While fingernails may feel hard and look waterproof, they're actually highly permeable. As nails absorb water, they swell; when they dry, they shrink. Repeat that cycle often enough—particularly in cold, dry weather, which also dries the nails—and they'll break or split at the ends.

Solvents, such as those in household cleaners, can also penetrate and chemically dry the nails. And activities like gardening and sports can break unprotected nails. Slamming your finger in a car door, along with other types of trauma to the base of the nail (the unseen portion beyond the cuticle), can cause permanent damage.

What passes for "nail care" can be a form of abuse. Various products, such as polish removers, can weaken the nails. An overly aggressive manicure can damage the nails. Worse, it can damage the cuticle, allowing infection to develop under the nail.

Infections can also fester in the gap between an artificial nail and the real nail. Wearing artificial nails longer than three months greatly increases that risk; so does regluing loose ones without using rubbing alcohol to clean them first.

PROPER CARE

Here are some basic steps you can take to ensure the health of your fingernails:

• Protect your nails from the ravages of water. Wear cotton-lined rubber gloves when doing household chores such as washing dishes.

• Immediately after exposure to water, apply an ordinary moisturizing lotion to your nails as well as to your hands.

• Wear gloves in cold weather and during activities that might harm your nails.

• Keep your nails short to help prevent breakage. Before trimming, soak them in water for a few minutes so they'll be less brittle under the clipper. File in only one direction—not back and forth, which can create splits. Apply moisturizer afterward.

• Don't pick at hangnails; that can break the skin and invite infection. Clip hangnails off close to the skin with cuticle scissors.

• Avoid nail-polish removers that contain acetone, which

can dry nails; look for ones that contain acetate instead. And use any remover as infrequently as possible.

- If you have your nails "done" professionally, make sure that sterile instruments are used. And ask the manicurist to be gentle on your cuticles.
- Don't turn to calcium, gelatin, vitamins, or other supplements to improve a nail problem. They won't.

The thyroid

THYROID MEDICATION AND HEAT

Q. *I have been taking Synthroid for thyroid disease for nearly ten years. About five years ago, I started getting very intolerant of heat. When the temperature rises over about 74° F, I become uncomfortably warm and begin to perspire. Recent tests show that my thyroid function is normal and that I'm not entering menopause. Could the medication be to blame?*

A. Heat intolerance from therapy with levothyroxine (*Levothroid, Synthroid*) usually results from overdosage. But since the dosage you're on apparently keeps your thyroid-hormone blood level in the normal range, that's unlikely to be the case. Nevertheless, you may be able to taper your dosage slightly (under your doctor's supervision, of course), relieve the heat intolerance, and still keep your test results in the normal range.

HYPOTHYROIDISM OR LAZINESS?

Q. *I used to be tired all the time, until doctors diagnosed a thyroid tumor. Before removing it, they started me on thyroid-hormone pills, which I continue to take every day. Almost immediately, my fatigue disappeared and hasn't returned. Is it possible that many people who are considered lazy actually have hypothyroidism?*

A. Not likely. Thirty or so years ago, thyroid hormone was the fashionable treatment for unexplained lethargy. Many people were unnecessarily "pepped up" with thyroid-hormone pills for years, often without a proper diagnosis of hypothyroidism (underactive thyroid gland). Today we know that hypothyroidism is not a common cause of chronic fatigue alone. There are usually other symptoms of hypothyroidism, including coarse scalp hair, intolerance to cold temperatures, constipation, dry skin, hoarseness, muscle cramps, and weight gain.

LONG-TERM THYROID THERAPY

Q. *In 1950, I was placed on thyroid-hormone therapy, and I've been taking 2 grains a day ever since. What are the likely consequences of such long-term medication?*

A. The medication is replacing what your own thyroid can't make. The adequacy of that dose can be verified by having your physician order a serum TSH (thyroid-stimulating hormone) level. Suppression of serum TSH below the normal range for many years can cause bone loss (osteoporosis), which could make you more vulnerable to fracture.

THYROID PILL DEPENDENCY?

Q. *I've taken a small dose of thyroid hormone every day for 40 years. My doctor hadn't diagnosed hypothyroidism; he just recommended the medication for chronic fatigue. Should I stop taking it?*

A. Probably. However, even though you may not have really needed the drug initially, your thyroid gland has adjusted to the supplement by decreasing its normal production of thyroid hormone. So if you go off the drug now, your thyroid gland could take up to six weeks to recover and you might suffer temporary symptoms of hypothyroidism, such as weight gain and sluggishness.

Still, it's better to avoid medication when your body can do the job itself. If you're willing to put up with those symptoms for a few weeks, talk to your physician about discontinuing the pills.

UNDERACTIVE THYROID?

Q. *According to information in a popular medical book, I may have an underactive thyroid gland. My hair, skin, eyes, and mouth are very dry; I have puffiness under my eyes, and I'm very sensitive to cold on my back. But a blood test indicates my thyroid is normal. Are there other ways I should be tested for an underactive thyroid?*

A. Not if you've had the two appropriate blood tests. One measures thyroid hormone itself, and one measures thyroid-stimulating hormone, or TSH. Your symptoms could be caused by many other problems, including dry environment, medical conditions that dry out the eyes, and certain skin diseases.

Water: diet and safety

MINERAL WATER SAFETY

Q. *The label on my brand of mineral water states: "Like other mineral waters, this should not be used as a sole source of drinking water." Is it safe to drink mineral water?*

A. Yes, but not liberally. Unlike bottled still water, mineral water is not tested and regulated by the FDA. Most mineral waters contain dissolved solids, sometimes even small amounts of toxic minerals such as arsenic. A daily glass or two shouldn't hurt you; but, as the label states, mineral water should not be your sole source of drinking water.

WATER AND DIETING

Q. *Some diet programs have you drink 10 glasses of water a day. What's the point?*

A. The main reason is to prevent kidney stones. Very-low-calorie diet programs can break down the body's protein stores, resulting in excess uric acid in the blood. When excreted in the urine, the excess acid can lead to kidney stones. Drinking large quantities of fluids dilutes the urine and lessens the likelihood of stones. In addition, drinking water frequently can stop hunger contractions of the stomach and create a temporary sensation of fullness.

WELL-WATER SAFETY

Q. *We recently moved to the country. Is well water automatically better for my family than city water, or can it be just as dangerous? Also, now that we're not drinking fluoridated water, what should I do to keep my family's teeth healthy?*

A. Well water is by no means automatically safer than city water. In fact, for well-run city systems supplied by protected reservoirs, the reverse may be true.

The quality of well water depends on what's in the underground aquifer from which it's drawn. Among potential aquifer pollutants are septic tank seepage, gasoline from leaking underground tanks, agricultural fertilizers and pesticides, road salt, and industrial wastes. To make certain your well is safe, have the water tested by a reputable laboratory. Your state health department might test your water for you, or suggest a lab to do so. Also check with your local water authority to determine whether periodic testing is advisable.

Make sure the initial test covers fluoride, which occurs naturally in some well water. Children under 14 need fluoride to strengthen their developing teeth. If your water doesn't have the optimal amount, your dentist or pediatrician can prescribe drops or chewable tablets. Using fluoridated toothpaste and fluoride rinses is sufficient to protect against tooth decay in most teenagers and adults.

Weight control

CAN DIET SODAS ADD WEIGHT?

Q. *I know diet sodas have few or no calories. But I seem to gain weight when I drink them. Could that be because they contain more sodium than regular soda and make me retain fluids?*

A. Diet soda isn't what's making you gain weight. That comes from eating too much or exercising too little. Many diet sodas do have more sodium than regular soda does. A 12-ounce can of *Diet 7-Up,* for example, contains about 70 milligrams of sodium, whereas regular *7-Up* has 32 milligrams.

But 70 milligrams isn't a lot. Since Americans consume about 2,300 to 6,900 milligrams of sodium a day, you'd have to guzzle lots of diet pop to boost your sodium intake significantly. Even if you did drink so much, the sodium wouldn't make your body retain a noticeable amount of fluid unless you had heart or kidney problems. People on sodium-restricted diets, however, probably shouldn't drink more than one or two cans of soda a day.

FLABBY ABDOMEN

Q. *How can a person lose fat from the lower abdomen when the rest of the body is relatively lean?*

A. There's no such thing as "spot reduction" exercises that zero in on fat in a specific area. When you work out, you use energy produced by burning fat from all over your body—not just around the muscles doing the most work. So aside from burning a few calories, all that exercises such as sit-ups do is strengthen your abdominal muscles and help hold your gut in.

However, studies do suggest that people losing weight—whether through any sort of exercise, calorie reduction, or both—tend to shed abdominal fat faster than fat from other parts of the body. That's good news, not only for your appearance, but also for your health: Abdominal fat seems to pose a higher risk of coronary heart disease than fat deposited in other areas.

MIDDLE-AGE SPREAD

Q. *What is the best way to control middle-age spread: diet, exercise, or both?*

A. Both—including exercises to tone muscles and burn fat. People acquire body fat in two distinct patterns. In so-called middle-age spread, fat accumulates in a "spare tire" around the belly, giving you an apple shape. The other distribution is pear-shaped, with fat deposited around the hips rather than the waist. Men are most often "apples"; women, most often "pears."

Exercises that strengthen your stomach muscles, such as sit-ups, can help restrain a bulging belly. But they won't reduce the amount of abdominal fat. The only way to take that fat off and keep it off is to eat fewer calories and do exercises like biking, jogging, swimming, and walking, which burn a lot of calories.

SKINNY PEOPLE, FATTY DIET

Q. *Since I'm very thin and want to gain weight, I eat plenty of fatty foods. Will my low weight keep my blood-cholesterol levels down despite the high-fat diet?*

A. No. A high-fat diet can increase blood-cholesterol levels in thin people as well as in heavy people. The body's tendency to convert dietary fat into blood cholesterol is entirely separate from its tendency to deposit that fat on your waist or thighs. To try to gain weight, increase your consumption of a variety of foods, not just fatty ones. But remember that thin people can have just as much trouble gaining weight and keeping it on as most heavy people do losing weight and keeping it off.

WHY THIN PEOPLE DON'T GAIN

Q. *Why do some people stay too thin even though they're trying to gain weight?*

A. Like their heavy counterparts, thin people seem to be programmed to remain close to a certain weight. They might be able to add pounds by cultivating patently unhealthy habits—avoiding exercise and gorging on high-calorie foods. But most thin people who tried to live that dieter's dream would actually find it hard to stay underactive and over-indulgent. Eventually, they'd revert to their usual habits and usual weight.

Thin people do have another option: muscle-building exercises. But again, the extra weight will be lost if they stop pumping iron.

Women's health

PAP SMEAR AFTER HYSTERECTOMY

Q. *My uterus was removed 24 years ago at age 36. All other reproductive organs were left intact. Since that time, I've received conflicting advice about the need to have an annual Pap smear when there's no uterus. Can you clarify?*

A. If your cervix was left in place when your uterus was removed, you definitely should still have an annual Pap smear to screen for cervical cancer. However, when the cervix is removed along with the uterus, there's no longer any need to have the test. While some doctors perform Pap smears even in those women to screen for vaginal cancer, that form of cancer is extremely rare and doesn't warrant an annual smear.

ANNUAL PAP SMEAR

Q. *How often should a woman get a Pap smear? And what time of month gives the most accurate results?*

A. The venerable Pap smear is one of the most important cancer-detection tests. A woman should begin having an annual Pap smear at age 18 (or earlier, if she is sexually active). Some gynecologists recommend that women at high risk for cervical cancer be tested even more frequently. (Risk factors include multiple sex partners, herpes simplex virus type 2 infection, and venereal warts.)

Pap smears should not be done during the menstrual period. Some recent data suggest that the test is more accurate during the first half of the cycle, if you use oral contraceptives. Midcycle is preferred for most other menstruating women.

Regardless of the timing, the technician reading the smear must know if you're taking oral contraceptives or estrogen replacement therapy, and the date of your last menstrual period.

ANTIBIOTICS AND YEAST

Q. *Every time I take antibiotics, I end up with a yeast infection. How can I prevent this?*

A. Whether or not yeast infections can be prevented is a matter of controversy. Since you always seem to get an infection when taking antibiotics, you could try using an antifungal vaginal cream at the same time. Those creams include butoconazole (*Femstat 3*), clotrimazole (*FemCare, Gyne-Lotrimin*), and miconazole (*Monistat 3*), all sold over the counter.

BREAST TENDERNESS

Q. *For breast tenderness, my gynecologist recommended 1,200 IU of vitamin E a day for life. He also recommended cutting back on caffeine. Are those treatments effective?*

A. There's no convincing evidence that eliminating caffeine or adding vitamin E helps relieve breast pain, which is usually caused by fluid retained just before menstruation. If your pain does precede menstruation, you might try taking a mild diuretic during the few days before your period. An over-the-counter pain reliever and a supportive bra might also help.

SOY AND BREAST CANCER

Q. *I have read that the plant estrogens in soybeans may not be safe for postmenopausal women. My oncologist "felt" that consuming soy was "probably" OK. But having had breast cancer, I don't want to follow feelings or "probablys."*

A. There's not enough hard evidence to make a definitive statement about the health effects of soy-based estrogens. Some observational studies have found that women who consumed the most plant-based estrogens have a lower risk of breast cancer than women who consumed the least. But there's also at least a theoretical concern that those compounds may stimulate tumor growth in women who have estrogen-responsive breast cancer, particularly postmenopausal women.

The overall pattern of your diet matters more than any one particular food. So we agree with Clare Hasler, Ph.D., a phytochemical researcher and executive director of the Functional Foods for Health program at the University of Illinois, who says it's OK for women—including postmenopausal women with breast cancer—to eat soy-based foods in moderate amounts as part of a balanced diet (low in animal fat, high in produce). But she would not recommend soy supplements until we know more about the health impact of high concentrations of soy compounds.

CONCERN ABOUT ABNORMAL PAP TESTS

Q. *My Pap tests have shown "slightly abnormal" cells for nearly two years now. Other than recommending more frequent testing, my doctors have not suggested any treat-*

ment. Recently I read in a newspaper column that "aggressive treatment" is necessary for premalignant stages of cervical neoplasia. What do you recommend?

A. Although "slightly abnormal" changes are not necessarily premalignant, you should nonetheless seek another opinion. Reasons for an abnormal Pap test result can range from vaginal or cervical infection to true cancer of the cervix. If the cause is an infection, treatment will usually lead to a normal Pap test; if not, the abnormality should be investigated further.

ESTROGEN AFTER HYSTERECTOMY

Q. *Four years ago, at age 30, I had a complete hysterectomy. After taking estrogen in several forms, I continue to have severe mood swings, hot flashes, depression, severe headaches, nervous conditions, and sharp pains in both of my breasts. Help!*

A. Your persistent hot flashes suggest that your dose of estrogen may be too low. Young women who have had a hysterectomy sometimes need more estrogen than older women going through menopause, in order to relieve the uncomfortable symptoms of abrupt hormonal decline. Your physician should work with you to find the dosage that is most effective.

ESTROGEN CREAM: HOW SAFE?

Q. *Would you comment on the possible adverse effects of estrogen in creams prescribed to treat vaginal dryness in postmenopausal women? Do they pose a risk to women with a family history of cancer?*

A. The risk is minimal. Although estrogen from those creams is absorbed into the bloodstream, no study to date has shown a health hazard from the use of vaginal estrogens. Most women will need to use the creams only about twice a week, which should be safe even if a woman has a family history of cancer. A woman who has had uterine or breast cancer herself, however, should not use estrogen in any form.

HOT FLASHES AND DIURETICS

Q. *I've heard that the water-ridding properties of diuretics such as* Dyazide *[triamterene/hydrochlorothiazide] make it essential to drink plenty of fluids during hot weather to prevent dehydration. Since the hot flashes that accompany menopause can also make you sweat, would that likewise lead to a dehydration risk from diuretics?*

A. No. Menopausal hot flashes are caused by temporarily dilated blood vessels in the skin. While that may make you sweat, you won't lose a significant amount of water, even if you're taking a diuretic.

HUNCHED BACK

Q. *I'm a 63-year-old woman and am starting to develop a hunched back. Is there some exercise to delay that?*

A. No. Your problem is probably osteoporosis, or bone thinning, which commonly follows menopause. The weakened spinal vertebrae simply fracture and collapse. You should consult your physician about the drug treatment options for osteoporosis, which include taking the female hormone estrogen (*Premarin*), alendronate *(Fosamax)*, raloxifene *(Evista)*, or the nasal spray calcitonin *(Miacalcin)*. Weight-bearing exercises, daily injestion of 400 to 800 I.U. vitamin D, and 1,200 milligrams elemental calcium should be basic treatment for osteoporosis.

ILLICIT DRUGS: PREGNANCY PERIL?

Q. *Ten years ago, in college, I experimented with several drugs, including marijuana, cocaine, and LSD. Now I'm 30 and my husband and I are thinking about starting a family. Have I done any permanent damage to my egg supply? Is the risk of birth defects increased?*

A. Go ahead and start your family. With the exception of certain anticancer medications, prior drug use, by males or females, does no appear to have any lasting effects on reproduction.

OSTEOPOROSIS AND THE PILL

Q. *From age 18 to 26 I had no menstrual periods. When my gynecologist prescribed birth-control pills a year ago, my menstrual cycle resumed. I've heard that lack of periods increases the risk of osteoporosis. Since birth-control pills contain estrogen, will they help reduce my risk?*

A. In your case, yes. Amenorrhea (the absence of periods) is usually associated with decreased production of the female hormone estrogen by the ovaries. Lack of estrogen can eventually lead to osteoporosis, which is characterized by less dense—and thus more fragile—bones. The birth-control pills are providing you with estrogen and helping prevent further bone loss. Women with normal periods already produce all the estrogen they need, so the Pill makes no difference to them.

An adequate calcium intake (at least 1,000 milligrams a day) and regular weight-bearing exercise before menopause can help build bone mass and protect against the chance of postmenopausal osteoporosis.

THE PILL AND BREAST CANCER

Q. *In your April 1999 issue, you mentioned that oral contraceptives can help reduce the risk of ovarian cancer and possibly uterine cancer and pelvic inflammatory disease. What effect does the pill have on the risk of breast cancer?*

A. Most studies have found no greater incidence of breast cancer among pill users. And in studies that indicated an added risk, that risk was too small to warrant that anyone stop taking the pill—even those who have a family history of breast cancer or a history of benign breast disease.

Oral contraceptives have also been associated with a greater risk of cardiovascular disease among women who have at least one cardiac risk factor, such as diabetes, high cholesterol, high blood pressure, smoking, or a family history of early coronary heart disease. For help in sorting out the risks and benefits of oral contraceptives, talk to your doctor.

OVARIAN CANCER CLUE?

Q. *I have heard on two television talk shows about a screening test for early diagnosis of ovarian cancer. What is the test and is it effective?*

A. A blood test called CA-125 is being used to monitor the treatment of women with ovarian cancer, and to check for recurrence. The test is very sensitive but not specific: It can detect ovarian cancer, but it also can turn up positive in the presence of other conditions, including pregnancy, endometriosis, uterine fibroids, and pelvic inflammatory disease. For that reason, many physicians do not use CA-125 as a screening test for ovarian cancer unless a woman is at high risk because of family history. Those women should have a CA-125 blood test annually, and should discuss with their physician the suitability of having an annual ultrasound examination of the ovaries.

POSTPARTUM DEPRESSION

Q. *What causes postpartum depression? What are the latest treatments?*

A. Postpartum depression—not the more common postpartum "blues"—is a psychiatric disorder that can severely impair day-to-day functioning. Its onset is usually within the first few weeks or months after childbirth. A woman who has once had postpartum depression can experience it again after future births.

The causes of postpartum depression are not well understood. The sudden change from the pregnant state, with accompanying changes in hormone levels, probably plays some role.

In contrast to the self-limited "blues," which usually lasts only a short time and needs only emotional support, true post-partum depression requires the attention of a psychiatrist. Antidepressant medications can help. Rarely, electroconvulsive (electric shock) therapy may be necessary.

Index